M000190924

Eating the *Shokuiku* Way

Eating the *Shokuiku* Way

The Japanese Guide to Raising Kids with Healthy Food Habits

Marie Akisawa and Motoko Kimura

ROWMAN & LITTLEFIELD
Lanham • Boulder • New York • London

Published by Rowman & Littlefield
An imprint of The Rowman & Littlefield Publishing Group, Inc.
4501 Forbes Boulevard, Suite 200, Lanham, Maryland 20706
www.rowman.com

86-90 Paul Street, London EC2A 4NE

British Library Cataloguing in Publication Information Available

Library of Congress Cataloging-in-Publication Data

Names: Akisawa, Marie, author. | Kimura, Motoko, author.
Title: Eating the Shokuiku way : the Japanese guide to raising kids with healthy
    food habits / Marie Akisawa and Motoko Kimura.
Description: Lanham : Rowman & Littlefield, 2022. | Includes index.
Identifiers: LCCN 2022023977 (print) | LCCN 2022023978 (ebook) |
    ISBN 9781538166536 (cloth) | ISBN 9781538166543 (ebook)
Subjects: LCSH: Cooking, Japanese. | School children—Food—Japan. |
    Food consumption—Health aspects—Japan. | LCGFT: Cookbooks.
Classification: LCC TX724.5.J3 A37 2022 (print) | LCC TX724.5.J3 (ebook) |
    DDC 641.5952—dc23/eng/20220803
LC record available at https://lccn.loc.gov/2022023977
LC ebook record available at https://lccn.loc.gov/2022023978

♾️™ The paper used in this publication meets the minimum requirements of
American National Standard for Information Sciences—Permanence of Paper for
Printed Library Materials, ANSI/NISO Z39.48-1992.

Contents

Chapter 1

Our Journey with *Shokuiku*

When Motoko was born, no one heard her cry. Winter held its breath outside the hospital windows in Kobe, Japan, as her mother heard doctors say frightening things like "She's weak," "Very small," and "She's too cold."

Her parents named her Motoko, which in Chinese characters means "energetic," hoping she'd gain strength and someday live up to her name.

She wouldn't make it easy. As an extremely petite child in kindergarten and elementary school, Motoko drove her mother crazy by barely eating. She got tired easily, and due to lack of energy, was indifferent to playing with other kids. But her mother, Toshiko (a high school health teacher and certified nutritionist who worked with over 6,000 students in her 25-year career), refused to give up on her.

Before dinner, as most Japanese families do, they clasp hands and practice a critical part of *Shokuiku*, called *Itadakimasu*. *Itadakimasu* means "I partake," and it is a spiritual thankfulness to the earth as well as all the people who worked to get food to our tables to nourish our bodies (figure 1.1).

After finishing dinner, Motoko's mother would serve her a rice ball. Though a tiny ball, little Motoko saw it as an insurmountable mountain of food. At the time, Motoko thought making her eat it was torture. Didn't her mother see she had no appetite? Motoko clamped her mouth closed and turned her face away from the food.

"Motokochang, the rice you ate at dinner was for your energy today and tomorrow. You need *this* rice now to get bigger and stronger." Motoko hated being the smallest in school, not able to reach things and constantly being teased as the classroom runt. So, she begrudgingly ate.

In time, Motoko's health and strength improved, and her height and weight reached the 50th percentile—happily average. Even more

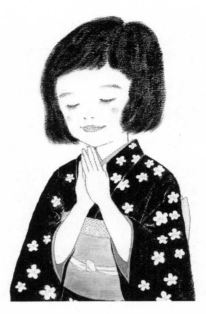

Figure 1.1   Itadakimasu

remarkable, she noticed an incredible increase in her ability to concentrate for abnormally long periods of time. For example, during the summer, Motoko had a stack of math and spelling books meant to take months of time to do. Instead of dragging it out, she decided she'd get it all done in one day so she could enjoy the rest of her summer. And she did! No problem. Ever since then, using the *Shokuiku* principles she's followed nearly her entire life, she can focus on a task undistracted for six to eight hours at a time.

Throughout Motoko's life in junior high and high school, her mom kept making rice balls for her. She prepared a bento box every day, and in it, Motoko had the most nutritious lunches.

"Bento box" is a Japanese term for a homemade lunch served in a container divided into sections, or "rooms," with each room being the home for an individual food. Think of a microwavable dinner tray, but instead of each compartment filled with processed, high-sodium, high-fat, high-sugar "food," each room inside a bento box is filled with fresh, wholesome fuel for your child's body (figure 1.2). With its colorful presentation, a bento box is quite beautiful to look at as well as alluring to eat!

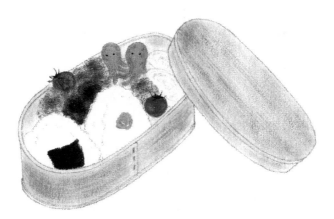

Figure 1.2   Bento Box

Diligent attention to nutrition allowed Motoko to achieve accomplishments greater than her peers. For example, she taught herself English and scored 109 on the TOEFL English test, the most recognized English test in the world. To put that score in perspective, most prestigious universities in America require at least a 68 on this exam, with Columbia requiring the highest score of 104+. That she could teach herself English and score that high on the exam is a testament to *Shokuiku* and food education.

With Motoko's mother's dedication to *Shokuiku*, and without ever having been told to study, Motoko got into one of the most prestigious universities in Japan, Sophia University, a top-five school (out of around 800), along with her friend and coauthor Marie, who had experienced a resurgence of health by eating the *Shokuiku* way.

Prior to getting into Sophia University, Marie experienced health problems after spending a year as an exchange student in San Antonio, Texas. There, she stopped practicing *Shokuiku* and started eating the "American way" (i.e., endless pizza, hot dogs, processed and fast foods with no concern as to where the food comes from [figure 1.3]). While she thought these addictive foods she enjoyed with her friends tasted great, her once-stellar grades and endless energy were replaced by lethargy, poor academics, lack of focus, weight gain, and depression. She felt her body shutting down on her. When she returned to Japan, she remembered *Shokuiku* and the way her mother would cook meals for her with fresh vegetables from nearby farms. In

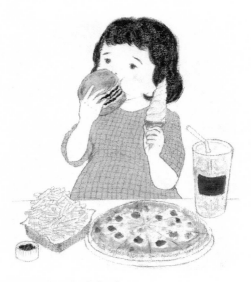

Figure 1.3   Eating American junk foods

desperation, Marie dedicated herself to going back to those ways. And guess what? Before long, her grades and health rebounded. She found her focus returned, her weight normalized, and her mental health improved. She also found her life mission—to help inspire others to eat this way.

In college, Marie and Motoko became best friends in their shared love for health and food. Marie shared that her father also had lapsed in his eating styles when he was an exchange student in the United States, and that may have caused him to develop type 2 diabetes in his 50s. To help improve the health of her father, and to avoid developing type 2 diabetes herself, Marie began to study nutrition and has become a registered dietician, and also a chef, and has learned a variety of healthy cooking techniques from traditional Japanese to macrobiotic.

After learning many types of cooking considered "healthy" in Japan, Marie realized that eating the *Shokuiku* way, the way her mother cooked for her every day when she was young, was the best way to stay healthy and energized after all. Special cooking techniques such as low-carb are critical for those who need special attention due to health conditions such as obesity and diabetes, but from the age of a toddler, it is important to eat as much of a variety of food as possible in moderate amounts following the *Shokuiku* way.

Marie has taught various healthy eating courses according to the needs of her students in Tokyo, and later decided to focus on low-carb cooking and started cooking daily for her father. Using her nutrition plan, her father reversed his type 2 diabetes in his 70s and is currently still working as an MD in his mid-80s, enjoying his energetic, long life with his beloved grandson. Marie became a gifted, sought-after registered dietitian, chef, and nutrition book author who serves as chairwoman of the Japanese Nutritious Foods Association, leading online courses on healthy eating.

Motoko went on to fulfill her dreams as a successful writer and movie producer, and after becoming a mother and traveling to America regularly, Motoko herself saw firsthand the damaging way Americans eat. Making things worse, every nanny she hired to help wasn't aware of the correct ways to feed a child. After experiencing this frustration, Motoko decided to spread the word about the benefits of raising kids the *Shokuiku* way.

***

Motoko's son attended an international Montessori preschool in Japan filled with students from all over the globe. She noticed students from Europe usually ate a lunch of pasta with butter, hard bread, and cheese from a paper bag. American students typically brought a peanut butter and jelly sandwich and an apple. Students from Africa ate fried chicken and potatoes; India students, curry and naan. Motoko had a chance to discuss *Shokuiku* with Eriko Jones, the school's director. Over the course of 24 years, Eriko has worked with over 2,000 students. Out of all the food cultures she's witnessed, the most impressive positive effects on learning have come from eating the *Shokuiku* way, which features diverse, colorfully balanced meals, including grains, vegetables, fish, and beans. *Shokuiku* can be practiced in any culture's food!

Also, Eriko noted that school lunches cut into bite-size pieces empowered and raised children's self-confidence by enabling them to eat easily and neatly on their own, fulfilling their need for independence (a.k.a. the "I Do It!" phase of childhood).

Students with brown, colorless paper-bag lunches filled with brown, somewhat nutrition-less foods sat next to students like Motoko's son with his bento box lunches filled with vivid, enticing foods. Her son's classmates asked him, "What is that?" "Is it good?" "Can I have some?" They'd try to sneak bites of his food! Vibrant and healthy lunches appeal to all children no matter their race or heritage. And they will appeal to your child as well.

Eriko noticed that students who brought colorfully balanced lunches could learn how to do complicated math such as division by the age of four compared to their classmates who did not.

***

Motoko is often asked, especially by American parents, how she gets her child to eat so adventurously or how she's maintained her own health and youth. In her late 40s, she still has to show identification to buy alcohol! Like her mother, she's never been hospitalized or significantly ill.

Right or wrong, parents tend to feed their kids similarly to how they grew up, and when faced with the challenge of changing this cycle for their own children, sometimes parents get a glazed look. After all, America is the birthplace of fast food, with over 66% of its population overweight or obese.[1] Everyone knows eating better is, well, better for us. But even though people know how important it is, they still go against what they know.

It can be challenging but not impossible to break this cycle.

***

A child is born with only half of his or her IQ genetically hardwired.[2] The rest is in our hands as parents to help our children achieve their best. We have only one shot at our children's formative years, and while we'll all make mistakes as parents along the way, the one thing we can make sure we do is set our children up for a long, healthy life.

Unlike the "tiger mom" stereotype you may associate with Asian mothers, Motoko's mother never pushed her too hard, but with her strong food foundation, Motoko blossomed on her own.

Motoko's ability to study improved due to practicing *Shokuiku* and consuming a nutritious balanced diet, consistently, every day.

Every meal is important. Having one balanced, nutritious meal once a week won't work. You need to care about what you and your child eat for every meal, one by one. And while *Shokuiku* takes some initial thought and effort, it is completely achievable and will become an easy way of life.

Shokuiku isn't a miracle switch where one day your child will suddenly become brilliant. But in order to put in the amount of effort needed to succeed, kids need the right energy and the highest-functioning brain possible. The correct foods help increase their concentration and allow them to awaken their full potential.

Motoko and Marie want to educate you and parents everywhere on the health benefits Japanese people have enjoyed for thousands of years, leading to Japan having the world's longest life span and lowest rate of obesity.

Motoko and Marie are here to make it easy. If you incorporate even a few *Shokuiku* principles into your family's eating lifestyle, you and your children will benefit. You picked up this book and you're well on your way!

Our goal with *Shokuiku* is to show how easy it is to adopt better eating principles. Through simple changes like serving your child a lunch in a bento box, which we will review in the following chapters, you can change your child's and your family's life. These *little* steps will lead to *big* changes in your family's health.

A QUICK BACKGROUND OF *SHOKUIKU*

Before we get into all the tips and tricks we'll be sharing throughout this book, it's important that we briefly explain the basics and background of *Shokuiku*.

The Basic Law of Shokuiku was enacted in Japan in 2005 as a way to tackle growing health issues that were popping up around the country. The idea of the law was to promote *Shokuiku* throughout Japan and get its citizens back on track with their health and nutrition. But *Shokuiku* was not a new concept in 2005. It originated in the late 1800s when many people in Japan were faced with nutrient deficiencies from poor diets. *Shokuiku* was born to teach these Japanese citizens about nutrition and help them improve their diets.

Shokuiku remains an integral part of life in Japan and has had a positive impact on the rates of disease, obesity, and longevity in the country.

The word *Shokuiku* translates to "food education," and while it does teach families about nutrition, it's much more than that. *Shokuiku* is made up of principles that parents follow when raising their children and teaching them how to eat properly. It's not a diet, but a way of life. The right nutrition knowledge can foster a healthy relationship with food. And when you have a good relationship with food, you also have the ability to respect your body, avoid crazy fad diets, maintain a healthy weight, and choose the best foods for your health for your entire life.

But *Shokuiku* is not just about teaching people how to eat for the most health benefits. It's also about connecting with the people and world around you. You'll learn in later chapters the importance of doing things like eating meals with your family as a way to bond, preparing foods with your kids, talking with your kids about food and culture, and showing gratitude toward food and the people that made it. It may not seem like it, but these types of actions go a long way in teaching kids about food, and even the world.

Chapter 2

Shokuiku for Babies and Toddlers

Can you imagine having a child who doesn't ask for sweets or who, after a few bites of ice cream, says, "Mom, I'm all done, it's too much"? This behavior is not a miracle. It is healthy conditioning using the practices of *Shokuiku* (figure 2.1). Motoko's seven-year-old son demonstrates this behavior consistently. Starting around age six, whenever he has been offered cake or candy, because of his solid *Shokuiku* conditioning, he self-regulates his body. He says, "Mommy, if I eat more of this, I'll get a stomachache."

Through *Shokuiku*, Motoko has taught her son how to listen to his body. She's given him the gift of moderation in a natural way, in a way that feels instinctual for him rather than someone "making him do it." The tools Motoko has given her son around food help ensure that it will be very unlikely for him to be faced with diet-related health issues down the road. And no matter the age of your children, it's not too late to give them these same tools.

THE *SHOKUIKU* FOUNDATION

In Japan, all parents learn *Shokuiku* when they prepare to have a baby. Just like Lamaze or Baby CPR classes taken in America, in Japan we take a class called *Shokuiku*, or "Food Education." The goal of this class is to teach parents the best way to feed their children to set them up for success. For example, Japanese parents learn that you can try to do a puzzle or sing the alphabet song to your toddler, but if all your child had to eat was pancakes with sugar-filled syrup for breakfast, he's not going to be able to sit still or absorb the information from his parents. Calorie-rich foods like pancakes and sugary syrup don't provide kids with the right nutrition to use

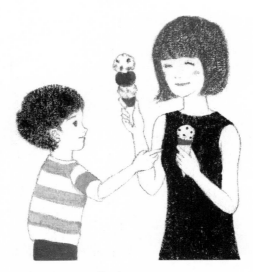

Figure 2.1   A boy choosing a smaller icecream

their brains to the full capacity (not to mention the fact that putting so much added sugar into a tiny body will make it hard for that body to remain still for any period of time!). Nutrient-rich foods are imperative for the brain to even have a shot at learning skills and information.

The people of Japan consider *Shokuiku* a basic way of life. They all learn the principles of this eating practice from day one of their lives and pass it down to their children and grandchildren. This is certainly not the way it is in the United States, but Americans can learn many things from the healthy ways of Japan and can start practicing *Shokuiku* no matter their age. Having the right nutrition education can help parents and kids make the best food choices throughout their lives that will help them achieve longevity.

In 1896, Dr. Sage Ishizuka (sometimes referred to as the "Vegetable Doctor") first discovered the connection between food and the aspects of aging and disease. He defined *Shokuiku* as the "scientific method to eat for longevity." You remember the scientific method, right? Dr. Ishizuka's mission was to help parents and children realize that learning how food is used in the body is the most important form of education, coming before academic study, before ethics, and even before exercise. **"Food education is the basis for *all* education,"** he said. And *Shokuiku* is the food education your family needs. According to the *Asia Pacific Journal of Clinical Nutrition*, "*Shokuiku* . . . cultivat[es] an ability to make choices about food;

fostering an understanding of traditional food culture; encouraging an attitude of respect for life and nature through food."[1]

The exceptional foundation of nutrition knowledge provided by *Shokuiku* helps Japanese people do so much more than just eat healthy foods. One concept of *Shokuiku* helps people feel more grateful and appreciative toward food, and this unlocks the door to many more health benefits. It may sound silly, but being grateful for your food will actually help you and your family have a better understanding of nutrition and where your food comes from, and this will promote better health outcomes.

When *Shokuiku* is a way of life during a child's early years, it is instilled deeply into their body and mind makeup. And when healthy habits are ingrained in this way, they will have an easier time bouncing back if they get off track over the course of their life. Remember Marie and her father's example of how they got their health back after going off-course in the first chapter? Both Marie and her father had lived in the United States during their high school years and indulged in the American way of eating—fast foods high in saturated fat and added sugars. It may have been fun at the time, but they both suffered the consequences with diabetes, weight gain, extreme lethargy, and all the complications that can come along with these issues. Once they connected how terribly they felt with their American eating habits, they went back to eating the *Shokuiku* way, and both were able to reverse major health problems within only one year. Of course, this was easy for them because they'd been raised in this way. But remember, it's not too late for your family. **Parents, it is critical you raise your children the *Shokuiku* way to make it easier for them to return to healthy eating over the course of their lives as well!**

FOOD QUALITY = LONGER LIVES FOR OUR CHILDREN

In America, parents typically focus their attention on what foods are "safe" and "unsafe" as they introduce foods into their babies' diet. New parents aren't taught to consider the quality of the food or how the food might translate into behavior, sleep habits, or life longevity. **American parents tend to seek convenience and quantity over quality,** and they typically feed their children the way they were raised, whether their upbringing was healthy or not.

Food quality, philosophy (teaching a healthy relationship with food), *and* offering a variety of foods (to avoid picky eating) are often overlooked in the critical first three years when your child is developing the most. This has partly led to the poor health statistics of Americans. The average life span of an American in 2020 was 77 years old, compared to 85 years old in Japan.[2]

Think about that: You could give (and get) the gift of an additional 10 years of life to your child by raising them to eat the *Shokuiku* way! Isn't that worth passing on some food items that give just momentary pleasure? If not for you, for your child, who is starting out in this world as a beautiful blank canvas and will think healthy food is delicious if you teach him or her to?

What American parents don't realize is this: The right quality foods can unlock the full potential of your child's mind and life span. "That's all? Food?" you might be asking. Yes, that's it! There is so much in parenting and health that is outside of our control, such as accidents and genetics. Don't you want to take control of the factors you can?

What you feed your baby will have a direct effect on how smart they become and how long they will live. And when we say quality foods, you probably already know what we're talking about. The foods with the best quality are those that offer the most nutrition. Quality foods are nutrient-dense, meaning they contain important macronutrients (carbohydrates, protein, and fat) and vital micronutrients (vitamins and minerals). Foods that are of a lesser quality will contain lots of things like sodium, added sugar, saturated fat, and empty calories that don't offer additional benefits. Examples of quality foods include, of course, fruits and vegetables but also whole grains, lean protein, and healthy fats. Foods that don't offer much in the way of quality include processed snacks, convenience meals, desserts, and fast food.

Kids absorb so much of what their parents teach them. If you feed your kids the best foods for their bodies from the start, you are laying an excellent foundation for their health for the rest of their lives. What you teach your child about food and nutrition will stick with them forever in one way or another. Kids who grow up in a healthy foods household are more likely to maintain healthy habits like eating fruits and vegetables once they are adults.[3] Parents only want the best for their kids, and healthy food choices are just that!

YOUR CHILD'S INTELLIGENCE AND
HEALTH IS DEPENDENT ON FOOD

Food can build or break down any human body, but the lifelong consequences of an unhealthy diet in the *first few years of life* are especially dire. It is widely supported that even mild nutrition shortages in the critical period of the first three years have a negative impact on a child's ability to thrive in intelligence, language, motor skills, and behavior.

Malnourished brains are smaller, have fewer neurons and synapses, and are challenged with other biological deficiencies. In fact, it's reported kids under three who are "food-insecure" (meaning healthy foods and quantity of foods not available to them) are:

- 90% more likely to have poorer health and
- 76% more likely to encounter problems with brain development in cognitive areas such as language and behavior.[4]

But even kids who aren't food-insecure aren't being fed the right foods to fuel their growing and developing brains. It may be surprising, but kids who eat plenty of food can also be malnourished. Babies, toddlers, and big kids need plenty of calories, protein, iron, healthy fats, vitamins, and minerals for their brains to grow to their full potential. A diet high in processed foods, let's say, may not provide much more than empty calories, sodium, added sugar, and saturated fat. The important nutrients needed for growing brains are severely lacking in convenience foods.

The journey to providing your children with the best foods for their brain actually starts in the womb when brain development begins. Unborn babies can be born malnourished if mom didn't eat properly during her pregnancy. This means pregnant mothers need to eat the same healthy calories and nutrients like protein, healthy fats, and micronutrients that babies and toddlers need.

A newborn's brain is only *one-fourth* the size of what their adult brain will be. In the first month of life, 100 billion brain cells multiply 20 times to make at least 1,000 trillion connections that we humans use to understand the world around us.[5] By your child's second birthday, her brain will be three-fourths of its adult size, and by her fifth birthday, her brain will be 90% of its adult size.[6]

Genetics account for about one-half of one's IQ.[7] The rest is environmental and up to us parents. What an opportunity to help shape your child's destiny!

Most doctors and scientists agree the first three years are a "critical period" where all of baby's senses are engaged—what she sees, hears, touches, smells, and tastes help shape how the brain thinks, learns, and feels.[8] Did you know that even the act of chewing increases blood flow to the brain?[9] But besides a baby's senses, good nutrition in the first three years of life can have a major impact on both life span and reducing the risk of many diseases in adulthood. **Basically, you can make a huge difference in your baby's intelligence, behavior, and health with how and what you feed your child in the first three years of life when their brain is doing most of its growing.**

As parents or parents-to-be, we dream of our kids growing up to be better, stronger, smarter, and faster than we are. We want to give them any edge we can to thrive in this increasingly competitive world. Feeding them the *Shokuiku* way will give them that edge.

BREASTFEEDING VS. FORMULA-FEEDING: BABY'S FIRST SIX MONTHS

If you're currently expecting a baby and considering whether you'll formula-feed or breastfeed, kudos to you for putting thought into that important decision. You've probably heard the saying "Breast is best." And while there are many advantages to choosing to breastfeed (such as the higher level of antibodies and cheaper cost), the saying should be "Fed is best" because it's most important that infants get enough calories and other nutrients to help them develop. Americans jumped on board the breastfeeding train around the 1970s. Prior to that, the convenience of formula-feeding reigned supreme. Now, about 56% of babies are breastfed until they're six months old.[10] And this is great because it is recommended that babies be breastfed or fed pumped breast milk for at least the first six months of life.

DHA (the type of healthy fat found in many fish like salmon and tuna) is one of the most important ingredients in breast milk or formula for a baby's overall growth and development. Because mothers in Japan tend to eat significant amounts of fish, the amount of DHA in their breast milk is higher than average. In fact, the amount of DHA in the breast milk of American women is about one-third of the breast milk in Japanese women, in fact.[11] You can always increase the amount of DHA and other important nutrients in your breast milk by improving your own diet. After all, what you eat as a nursing mother directly affects your little one (in both positive and negative ways).

Breastfeeding or pumping is not an option for all mothers. Sometimes it just doesn't work and there can be many reasons why this is so. Fortunately, formulas these days contain the important nutrients your baby needs to grow. Like breast milk, formula will give your baby the energy, hydration, and key vitamins, minerals, and macronutrients they need. Formula is made to mimic breast milk as closely as possible. This means you can find formula options with high amounts of nutrients like DHA and other healthy fats, probiotics, and proteins.

BEGINNING SOLIDS, THE *SHOKUIKU* WAY

According to the American Academy of Pediatrics, by about six months you can start to consider solid foods for your baby, in addition to breast milk or formula up to 12 months of age.[12] But please check with your child's pediatrician first to get the official solid-foods green light!

The biggest difference between traditional American baby feeding and the *Shokuiku* method is that parents in Japan don't use *any* processed food for the first few months of solid feeding. Babies' new stomachs need to start with *fresh* foods, like unflavored veggies, fruits, and grains (figure 2.2). This ensures they can learn how food should truly taste. They need to learn what a carrot, pea, or squash tastes like without any extra flavors, spices, or sweeteners. Parents sometimes put their own tastes in the forefront and

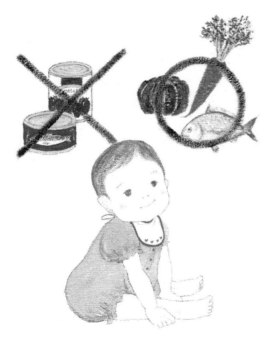

Figure 2.2   Baby eating only fresh foods.

Table 2.0 *Shokuiku* Food Introduction Chart

Age	Development Guidelines	Frequency	Milk	Consistency	Estimated Amount of Food per Serving
6 months	Keep an eye on baby—ensure they can close mouth and swallow prior to beginning solids.	Once a day	After giving new ingredient of baby food, also offer previous foods they've tried. What to offer or the amount can be managed by seeing how the baby is coming along. Then follow with as much breast milk or formula as baby wants.	Smooth, mashed, or ground	One spoonful of one ingredient at a time and nothing processed. Try two new ingredients a week. For example: 1. Grains (start with rice, boiled and smashed). 2. Veggies (mashed) like potatoes and carrots. 3. Fruits (mashed) like fresh apples, bananas, and watermelon without seeds. 4. Fish (once baby gets used to eating baby food, try feeding ground white-fleshed fish). 5. Chicken (ground, cooked). 6. Pork (ground, cooked). 7. Tofu / egg yolk (ground, cooked). 8. Beef (ground, cooked) and soft dairy products like plain yogurt without sugar.

Age	Ability	Frequency	Instructions	Texture	Amounts
7–8 months	Always supervise your baby while they eat. Milk teeth start to grow. Able to grind food with tongue and upper jaw.	Twice a day	After giving the new ingredient of baby food, offer previous foods they've tried. Then follow with as much breast milk or formula as baby wants about three times a day.	Soft enough so baby can grind food with their tongue	Keep moving down the list of foods, making sure they are smooth and ground in texture. Increase the variety of food after each one is introduced so baby can enjoy the tastes and feelings on the tongue. Grains: 50–80g Veggies and fruits: 20–30g Fish: 10–15g Chicken, beef, or pork: 10–15g Tofu: 30–40g Egg: 1 yolk (avoid whites for now) Dairy: 50–70g
9–11 months	Able to grind food with their gums	Three times a day Baby should experience the joy of eating together with others.	After giving baby their solid food, give as much breast milk or formula as baby wants, about two times a day.	Soft enough so baby can grind food with their gums	Grains: 90g Soft rice or pasta: 80g Veggies and fruits: 30–40g Fish: 15g Chicken, beef, or pork: 15g Tofu: 45g Egg: 1/2 egg Dairy: 80g

(continued)

Table 2.0 (Continued)

Age	Development Guidelines	Frequency	Milk	Consistency	Estimated Amount of Food per Serving
12–18 months	At around 1 year old, all 8 front teeth may be in, and in the latter half of this time period, molars will start to grow and baby will start using their teeth.	Three times a day Begin to regulate the meal schedule in baby's daily life. Encourage baby to grasp their food and enjoy the eating experience.	After offering solid food, give baby breast milk or formula as they desire.	Soft enough that baby can chew food with their gums	Grains: 90g Soft rice or pasta: 80g Veggies and fruits: 40–50g Fish: 15–20g Chicken, beef, or pork: 15–20g Tofu: 50–55g Egg: 1/2–2/3 egg Dairy: 100g

Table 2.1 *Shokuiku* Food Introduction for 5- to 18-Month-Olds

	Foods	5–6 months	7–8 months	9–11 months	12–18 months	Memo
Grains	Rice	●	●	●	●	
	Oatmeal	●	●	●	●	Boil water and turn down the heat to medium-low and cook the oats for 5 minutes, until all of the water is gone and the oats are soft.
	White bread	●	●	●	●	1. Cut off bread crust and tear bread in small pieces. 2. Smash 1 adding water. 3. Bring to a boil and cool it to serve.
	Pasta	✕	▲	●	●	Make sure you simmer well so the texture becomes mushy.
	Corn flakes	✕	▲	●	●	Cook well until it becomes soft enough for the baby.
Veggies	Carrot	●	●	●	●	Highly nutritious with carotenoids.
	Pumpkin	●	●	●	●	Peel the skin for 5–8 months old, and if you simmer until soft, with skin is okay from 9 months old.
	Potato, sweet potato	●	●	●	●	Easy to smash, filled with vitamin C.
	Tomatoes	●	●	●	●	Peel off skin and get rid of seeds.
	Spinach	●	●	●	●	Simmer well, and scum (bitterness) should be skimmed.
	Turnip, radish	●	●	●	●	Turnip gets softer when simmered.
	Onion	●	●	●	●	Onions get sweeter as they are heated.
	Cabbage, bok choy	●	●	●	●	Plenty of vitamin C.

(continued)

Table 2.1 (Continued)

	Foods	5–6 months	7–8 months	9–11 months	12–18 months	Memo
	Broccoli, cauliflower	●		●	●	Babies can also use their hands to eat them.
	Pepper, paprika	×	▲	●	●	Start from after 9 months old since they are a little hard to smash.
	Okra	×	●	●	●	Mince well, and you'll be able to add thickness.
	Eggplant, cucumber	▲	●	●	●	Start from about 6 months old when baby begins to get used to eating veggies.
	Various mushrooms	×	×	▲	●	Mince well since mushrooms are hard to chew because of high fiber content.
Fruits	Apples	●	●	●	●	Regulate the functions of intestines.
	Bananas	●	●	●	●	Mash to a paste.
	Raisins	×	×	▲	●	Dry fruits should be simmered and minced into small pieces.
	Kiwi	×	▲	●	●	Acidity can be a burden to baby's stomach so need to pick fully ripened kiwi from after 9 months old.
	Strawberries	×	▲	●	●	Acidity can be a burden to baby's stomach so need to pick fully ripened strawberries from after 9 months old.
Protein	Tofu	●	●	●	●	Start with Kinugoshi and then Momen.
	White-fleshed fish	●	●	●	●	High protein, good for digestion.
	Egg	●	●	●	●	Start with yolk and then whites.
	Natto (fermented soybeans)	▲	●	●	●	Highly nutritious food, good for digestion.

					Notes
Yogurt	▲	●	●	●	Yogurt with no sugar is a must.
Cheese	X	▲	●	●	Cottage cheese from 9 months and processed cheese from 12 months.
Milk, soybean	X	▲	▲	●	It's okay to simmer and use it with cooking, but baby needs to be older than 1 year old to drink it.
Chicken	X	●	●	●	Start in the order of minced chicken, chicken breast, and chicken thigh.
Beef, pork	X	▲	●	●	Start in the order of chicken, beef, and pork.

Key:
● = recommended
▲ = okay to give but could wait
X = not recommended

think, "That sounds so boring," but keep in mind how new your baby's tongue is. You don't need to add any salt, sugar, or additives to your baby's first foods. *Any* new flavor is going to be huge and exciting!

Tables 2.0 and 2.1 will be a guideline, but keep in mind you must look for signs for your baby's food readiness (good neck control, reaches for food, no longer pushes food out of her mouth with her tongue, wants to chew). You should adjust how and what you offer according to your child's development, growth, and appetite. All kids develop at different paces!

Homemade Food vs. Prepackaged Food

While store-bought baby food offers the fastest solution for feeding babies, many brands include ingredients that should be avoided in the first year of life (like sugar and salt).

For the highest quality, safety, and nutrition, it's always best to prepare food yourself by boiling, cooking, and mashing. When you make your baby's food all yourself, you get to control exactly what is in it and there is no mystery in what your tot is eating. Interestingly, one study showed that by 12 months old, babies who were fed homemade baby food had a healthier body weight than other infants.[13]

Motoko, being a working mom herself as a producer in the film industry with a heavy travel schedule, understands completely why sometimes buying ready-made jars is most convenient. Because she didn't want to use prepackaged foods with her son, she would make batches of homemade soft foods at a time and keep them in the refrigerator for up to a week or in the freezer for longer. If you're also a busy parent, you can do this by dedicating just an hour a week to meal prepping your little one's food.

When babies are first starting solid foods, it's recommended that they try just one flavor at a time. This cannot only help eliminate any possible food allergies but also help your baby learn and enjoy many different flavors of foods. Eating mixed flavors too soon can mask the true flavor of foods a baby is eating, and this could cause some picky eating habits down the road. This can especially be true of baby foods that have been flavored with unnecessary additives.

If you go the premade route, look for options made from whole foods and that don't include harmful ingredients like salt and sugar. Not only do these ingredients mask flavors that you want your baby to learn to love, but they also can harm your baby's development. Not to mention that a few years later, when your baby is no longer a baby and is still eating lots of processed foods and added sugar, this could affect his attention span at school. How will a five-year-old ever enjoy fresh green beans if the beans they were fed as an infant were masked with salts and other flavors? A key part of *Shokuiku* is teaching children appreciation for the food in its whole, natural form.

Some parents get nervous about feeding their baby fish during the first year, because mothers were trained not to eat much tuna during pregnancy due to mercury levels. But low-mercury fish should be part of every child's diet if possible. It is now proven that eating fish aids with development, as well as improving children's IQ scores and sleep.[14] Yes, sleep! Besides fish, you can even give your infant other common allergens when starting solid foods, like peanuts, eggs, and wheat.

In a nutshell, babies just don't need many of the foods American adults are used to eating. Not only that, but certain foods can be harmful to a baby's development and can cause issues later in life. Laying down a good foundation of nutrition now with your baby will likely lead to a life of making proper food choices. And isn't that exactly what you want as a parent, to teach your kid how to make the best decisions in life?

With this in mind, it's important to point out the foods that should be avoided in the first year of life when practicing *Shokuiku*. These foods won't do anything positive for your baby's health. Instead, unfortunately, they will just add unnecessary and harmful ingredients to his tiny, growing body.

Common foods to avoid during baby's first year to practice *Shokuiku*:

- Ketchup
- French fries
- Pancakes and syrup
- Sugary yogurt and yogurt drinks
- Snack puffs filled with sugar

THE FIVE SENSES

Before you start enrolling your baby or toddler in every learning class you can find from music to baby gymnastics, you need to feed them correctly and teach them how to eat. Otherwise, all the learning they get in those classes won't be retained!

When your child is eating the *Shokuiku* way, they're exposed to a bevy of education just by eating and sharing meals with you. There isn't a toy in the world that can give your child an all-five-senses learning experience. And food is the best lesson in the five senses.

Think about your favorite meal from your favorite restaurant. No matter what it consists of, it is a complete sensory experience. **You see the colors** on your plate: reds, greens, browns, yellows. **You smell the delectable aromas** of your cuisine wafting into your hypothalamus that stimulates hunger (you know that feeling when you walk past an Italian restaurant and the smell of garlic makes you want to eat right then and there?). **You hear the crunch** of a cucumber bite from a fresh salad. **You touch the textures** of finger foods as you lift them to your mouth. **And of course, taste.** If you close your eyes and take a moment as you chew, think of how many flavors you can taste from sour to sweet to savory.

Incorporate play and narration and fun into meals with your child, using the five senses as your guide. Ask your child if what they smell reminds them of any other food they've eaten and join them! Babies and children learn how to eat and feel by mimicking you (figure 2.3).

- **Describe what shapes, colors, and sizes you see on your plates.** For example, say, "Look how broccoli looks like the forest!" or "Can you see how these diced cheese cubes can be stacked like building blocks?"
- **Narrate how the food sounds as they chew and bite it.** "Do you hear how that carrot snaps in your teeth? It sounds like a stick breaking, doesn't it? Fun! Let's snap some more sticks!"
- **Let your child feel and play with their food,** exploring it with their mouths and hands, so they can learn about textures and get comfortable with everything from smooth foods to clumpy, slippery ones.

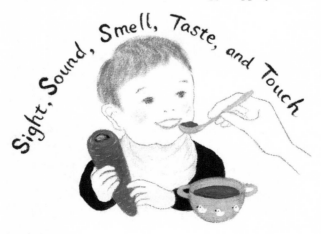

Figure 2.3   Five Sences

• **Ask your toddler to relate foods to each other.** Do green beans taste like asparagus? Do oranges taste like bananas? This can be a very fun time at the table bonding with your child and creating a positive association with food on top of encouraging them to enjoy it.

Making food a fully sensory experience entices children into eating and enjoying healthy foods. Eating this way helps children develop their senses and their vocabulary, builds skills in categorizing and observing, teaches cause and effect, and most importantly, is just plain fun!

MORE SHOKUIKU FEEDING TIPS FOR BABY'S FIRST YEAR

We'll cover plenty of tips, tricks, and facts about feeding your kids throughout this book. But since we are mostly talking about the first year of life here, let's look at a few more points:

• Offer a new ingredient every week. When you do this, you will quickly expand your child's palate and set them up for less picky eating habits once they hit toddlerhood.
• Incorporate seasonal foods. You'll soon learn how seasonal fruits and vegetables reign supreme and can offer the biggest nutrition punch for babies and kids of all ages (and even parents!).
• When starting "real food," make it small, for the purpose of choking prevention and so children can eat without making a mess (before 18 months old, though, let them make a mess!). Feeding themselves will build the confidence they can do it on their own.
• Keep it simple: If you don't want to make your own baby food, premade is fine, just make sure it's not ultra-processed and is made without extra flavors and additives.
• Be careful of the sneaky ways sugar gets into toddlers' diets (check labels!).

SHOKUIKU AND CHILDCARE

One of the inspirations for writing this book occurred when Motoko traveled to the United States during her son's young childhood, and while she worked she hired babysitters and nannies to help watch him. She noticed how inexperienced American childcare providers were with the style in which she wanted her son to continue eating.

It can feel daunting to provide instructions to grandparents, nannies, and other people who don't know much about nutrition. To make things a bit easier, here are some tips for working with your child's caregiver to help incorporate *Shokuiku*:

- Freeze homemade foods or meals that can be easily reheated. This makes it easy for a caregiver to feed your child the foods you want them to be eating.
- Let the caregiver know which snacks (if any) are appropriate for your child to eat while you are away.
- Preapprove all restaurants and take-out places, as well as menu items, to which your caregiver is allowed to take your child.
- It is always best to pack premade food and snacks if the caregiver will be taking your child out of the house.

If you have challenges getting caregivers (especially ones you're not employing, like grandparents) to incorporate *Shokuiku*, try sharing with them the main concepts of what you're trying to do and why you are trying to get their support. You can always use this book as a resource! And don't be afraid to send food you want your child to eat at their house. You are the parent!

SHOKUIKU OVERVIEW OF THE FIRST YEAR

1. **Breastfeed if possible,** and if you formula-feed, look for high DHA content.
2. **Introduce foods one at a time** to baby, including fish when the time is right (see table 2.1), and avoid all spices and sugar so baby can appreciate the full flavor of each food.
3. **Continue introducing new flavors** with whole foods (no additives!) to expand your baby's palate.
4. **Make feeding times fun!** Narrate what's on your baby's plate.
5. **Incorporate the five senses** to engage baby's brain and enjoyment, which aids in development and a healthy joy of eating!
6. **Eat with baby** when you can so they can "feed" off your enjoyment and appreciation for the healthy foods on your plate.

Chapter 3

Smarter Children = Smarter Adults

Small children, especially those who have not grown up the *Shokuiku* way, cannot be expected to make healthy food choices on their own. Once they're in preschool especially, and begin to be influenced by other children and the food around them, many children will pick French fries over carrots, or a sweet muffin over a plain egg. They aren't mature enough to know how the wrong foods can damage their bodies. A preschooler cannot yet connect the way they feel after a meal with what they actually ate.

As adults, *we* know, for example, that if we eat a double cheeseburger, fries, and a milkshake at lunch, we may feel sluggish later in the afternoon. As adults, that is our choice. But kids—our precious, naive kids—unless they are taught, have *no idea* about the repercussions of what they put in their bodies and how it affects their mood, sleep, focus, energy level, and especially how long they'll live. They need you to guide them and provide nutritious foods every day!

You can prevent your kids from growing up to be obese and unhealthy. Don't you think it's a necessity to set your kids up for a long life?

UNLOCK YOUR CHILD'S HEALTH IN THREE STEPS

We've come up with three simple steps that you can do every day to improve your child's health. We promise they're easy! And we're not talking about anything that will require too much of your precious time either.

Bento boxes are widely used in Japan and are easy to mimic. They're perfect for school lunches, which are notoriously unhealthy in America (more on that later). We'll be giving you plenty of ideas for ways to fill your child's bento box for school lunches or other meals.

All you have to do to get started is:

1. **Buy a bento box,** available at many housewares stores as well as online.
2. **Fill it with healthy foods** to turbo-power your child's brain.
3. **Do this every day!** Consistency is key to results. We know that environmental influences on a child's IQ have to be done persistently to be effective.[1]

Don't worry, we'll make it easy! **With the right ingredients on hand, making a bento box should only take you 10 minutes a day.** You already have to make *something* for your children to eat, why not put in food that will help them thrive?

BENTO BOXES

Perhaps you've ordered a bento box at a restaurant or seen it as a social media fad, but in Japan, bento boxes are a regular part of everyone's— adults and kids—daily life.

The first use of bento boxes can be traced back to the late 1500s, when people put food in lacquered boxes to enjoy while having tea and viewing cherry blossoms (*Hanami*).[2] Then, people started bringing "rice bowls" wrapped up in leaves to carry food to work. In modern times, parents most often make bento boxes for their children's and their own lunches.

Bento boxes help ensure children are getting all of the nutrients they need to develop. *Bento* means "useful thing" or "convenience." It is a dish, tray, or box that is split up into compartments (or in Japan we call them "rooms") that can be filled with a variety of well-portioned, nutrient-rich foods.

The most helpful thing about bento boxes for parents is that they make healthy lunch-making easy. All you have to do is assign each compartment, or "room," in the tray a food label so you can easily keep track to make sure your child is getting the full nutrition they need. There will be the protein room, the vegetable room, and the carbs room. This way, you can see what your child is eating and if they have enough of the key foods they need. You can rest assured that you have packed not too much or too

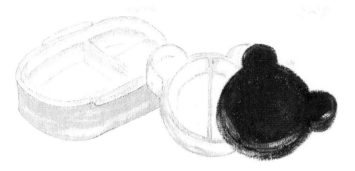

Figure 3.1　Bento Boxes

little, but the perfect amount of food, using the premeasured spaces in the box.

You can find bento boxes everywhere, in retail stores or online. They come in all shapes and sizes, from round to rectangle, and some with thermal protection for packing soups as well. They even license popular children's characters your child may love (figure 3.1). And they can increase in size as your child gets older.

But you don't have to buy a special bento box to utilize *Shokuiku*. You can group together any small, reusable containers for the compartments you need. The key is knowing how much you are feeding your child and how many different kinds of nutritious foods. Aim for at least four different ingredients of food in each box.

Bento boxes not only are the easiest way to get your children to be attracted to the food you want them to eat, but also help parents make sure they're covering their bases on offering a wide variety of healthy foods. Their presentations can be so colorful, almost like pieces of art, that kids can't wait to open them up and dig in!

In your bento box strategy, **assign each compartment a type of food** to help you make sure your child is getting enough protein and healthy carbohydrates for energy. It is not just talk—protein, healthy carbs, and micronutrients (vitamins and minerals) are essential to a child's growth. Children need nutrients like protein, vitamins, and fatty acids to build tissues that develop their brains.[3] A lack of these important nutrients increases the risk of neurological and psychiatric disorders and can also lead to delays in physical growth.[4]

So, now that you're ready to start using bento boxes to help tackle your child's health, below is an example template of how you can arrange each "room" of a bento box. Each section should be cut into approximate thirds, with fruits and snacks served on the side.

$$1/3 = \text{Protein}$$

$$1/3 = \text{Veggies}$$

$$1/3 = \text{Carbs}$$

BEST BENTO BOX FOODS AND WHY THEY'RE AMAZING

There are numerous types of healthy proteins, veggies, and carbs that you can use to fill the "rooms" of your kid's bento box—so much so that they could easily eat something new every day! And variety is what it's all about. Introducing your kids to different foods and nutrients regularly can help them be less picky eaters while also improving their health.

Let's look at some ideas for foods to put in bento boxes and how they are packed with nutrition. Don't forget to get creative and switch things up here and there!

Protein

Hardboiled eggs: Research suggests that choline in eggs is critical for infant development and brain function.

Ground beef: Ground beef and other meats are soft and easy for kids to chew.

Tofu: Tofu not only is a great plant-based protein source but also contains antioxidants that can work in your child's body to ward off illnesses. There are many ways to prepare tofu to make it interesting and fun to eat.

Bacon: Bacon can be easily rolled along with veggies like asparagus or enjoyed with peas.

Cheese: A good, filling source of protein that happens to taste great with practically any veggies.

Salmon: Astaxanthin is an antioxidant found in salmon that may benefit heart, brain, nervous system, and skin health. Salmon is one of the best sources of the omega-3 fatty acids, EPA and DHA, that help decrease inflammation, lower blood pressure, reduce the risk of cancer, and improve heart health.

Fruits and Vegetables

Tomatoes: Tomatoes contain key antioxidants like lutein and lycopene, two types of carotenoids. These can protect the eyes against light-induced damage.

Eggplant: The antioxidants, anthocyanins and chlorogenic acid, found in eggplant protect cells from damage caused by free radicals.

Baby corn: While corn is famous for its high starch and carb content, baby corn is less starchy. It has plenty of fiber and protein and is the perfect size for kids!

Broccoli: Broccoli is high in many nutrients, including a family of plant compounds called isothiocyanates. "Isothiocyanates" may be impossible to say, but they reduce oxidative stress and lower the risk of neurodegenerative diseases.

Bell peppers: Bell peppers are excellent sources of vitamins A and C, potassium, folic acid, and fiber. Did you know bell peppers actually contain more vitamin C than oranges?

Asparagus: Asparagus is packed with antioxidants, helping to neutralize cell-damaging free radicals. It's also a great source of fiber, a key nutrient to keeping your little one from getting backed up.

Blueberries: Blueberries contain an important nutrient, anthocyanin. Anthocyanin gives blueberries their deep blue color as well as many of their health benefits including antioxidant activity and anti-inflammatory effects, two factors important to keeping a healthy heart.

Edamame: Edamame is rich in protein, antioxidants, and fiber that may lower circulating cholesterol levels. It is also rich in vitamin C.

Pumpkin: Pumpkin is high in vitamins and minerals while being low in calories. It's also a great source of beta-carotene, a carotenoid that your body converts into the vitamin A you need for the health of your eyes, skin, and immunity.

Okra: Okra is rich in antioxidants that may reduce your and your child's risk of serious diseases, prevent inflammation, and contribute to overall health. Most notably, it contains polyphenols (another antioxidant) that may contribute to heart and brain health.

Strawberries: A great source of vitamin C, strawberries also provide plenty of fiber, potassium, and antioxidants.

Carbs

Carbohydrates are necessary for a child to have enough energy to get through the day. There are many types of carbohydrates, and it can get downright confusing when trying to figure out which ones are best to eat. Whole grains are the most nutritious carbohydrate option. This is because whole grains are minimally processed and contain lots of fiber, minerals, B vitamins (like folate, niacin, and thiamine), antioxidants, and even some protein. Eating more whole grains has been linked to lower risks of heart disease, diabetes, and obesity, especially when compared to enriched grains, like those used to make white bread, baked goods, and processed snacks.

Carbs are also sometimes called sugars. However, there are two types of sugars to be aware of. Natural sugars are found in fruits and don't have the same effect on your blood sugar as added sugars. Besides this, fruits contain so many other important nutrients that make them a vital part of an overall healthy diet. But when you see added sugars on a nutrition label, these are much different than natural sugars. Added sugars are often found in processed foods, desserts, and sweet cereals and drinks. These sugars go by many names, like dextrose, fructose, corn syrup, and cane juice. It's best to limit or avoid added sugar and do your best to stick to foods that contain *natural* sugars, like fruit.

Examples of healthy carbs to include in a bento box include:

- Brown or wild rice
- Whole-grain crackers
- Whole-grain pasta
- Whole-grain bread, tortillas
- Oats
- Quinoa
- Any type of fruit—the more variety, the better!
- Starchy vegetables like baked potatoes or sweet potatoes (not French fries—these contain too many calories and the oil they are prepared in can go rancid!), peas, beans, chickpeas, and lentils

BENTO BOX RECIPES

Ready to get started making your first bento box? Here are some beautiful and savory recipes that will delight your child!

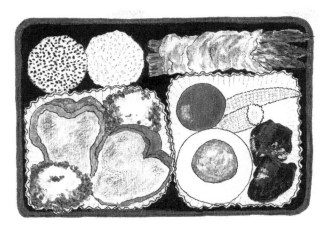

Figure 3.2 Bento 1

Stuffed Peppers, Rice Balls, and Veggies (figure 3.2)

Ingredients:

4 ounces Japanese short-grain white rice plus 4 ounces water (can make
  5–6 small rice balls)
Black and white sesame seeds (handful total)
1 egg
Salt
1/2 red bell pepper
1/2 green bell pepper
Raw ground beef to stuff in each pepper, about a large meatball size
1 tablespoon grated Parmesan cheese
2 stalks asparagus
2 strips raw bacon
2 pieces broccoli
1/4 eggplant
1 piece baby corn
Olive oil
1 cherry tomato

Instructions:

1. Cook rice for rice balls. After rinsing rice, put rice and water in a saucepan and before you cook it, let it sit for about 20 minutes with no heat. Heat rice (in water) until it comes to a boil, then lower the heat with a lid on. Simmer until the water is almost gone and rice becomes soft and sticky. If the rice gets too soft, you can microwave it for about a minute, so it will be easy for you to make rice balls with it. After making two rice balls, sprinkle them with white and black sesame seeds.
2. Boil the egg for 10 minutes, then cut it in half. Sprinkle with a little bit of salt.
3. Stuff each pepper with raw ground beef mixed with Parmesan cheese. Make sure to mix beef well with cheese.
4. Cut each asparagus stalk into three pieces and cut each strip of bacon into three pieces. Roll the asparagus pieces with the bacon pieces.
5. Put broccoli, eggplant, baby corn, stuffed peppers, and asparagus-bacon rolls on a baking tray. Sprinkle a pinch of salt or Parmesan cheese and drizzle olive oil over the top. Cook in the oven for 10 minutes at 350 degrees Fahrenheit.
6. Place everything plus the tomato in a bento box.

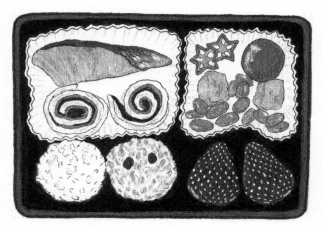

Figure 3.3   Bento 2

Omelet, Rice Balls, Veggies, and Fruit (figure 3.3)

Ingredients:

4 ounces Japanese short-grain white rice plus 4 ounces water (can make
  5–6 small rice balls)
1 egg, beaten
Salt
2 tablespoons cooked ground beef
Ketchup
1 slice salmon
Olive oil
1 thin slice ham
1 piece seaweed
2–3 pieces cubed pumpkin
1 piece okra
12–14 edamame beans, shelled
1 cherry tomato
2 strawberries

Instructions:

1. Cook rice for rice balls. After rinsing rice, put rice and water in a
   saucepan and before you cook it, let it sit for about 20 minutes with
   no heat. Heat rice (in water) until it comes to a boil, then lower the
   heat with a lid on. Simmer until the water is almost gone and rice
   becomes soft and sticky. If the rice gets too soft, you can microwave
   it for about a minute, so it will be easy for you to make rice balls with
   it.
2. Scramble half of your egg mixture. Make one rice ball with the
   scrambled egg and a bit of salt. Make another rice ball with the cooked
   ground beef and a bit of ketchup.
3. Lightly sauté salmon in olive oil.
4. Fry the second half of the egg mixture and make a thin omelet by roll-
   ing up the egg with the ham and a piece of seaweed in it. Cut in half.
5. Boil or steam pumpkin and okra with a pinch of salt.
6. Place everything into a bento box with edamame beans, a cherry
   tomato, and strawberries.

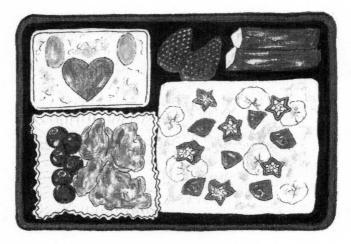

Figure 3.4 Bento 3

Protein-Rich Open-Faced Sandwich, Chicken, and Fruit (figure 3.4)

Ingredients:

Small handful shredded cheese (mozzarella has the lowest sodium)
3 shrimp, diced
1 large cherry tomato, diced
1 okra, diced
1/4 red bell pepper, diced
Real mayonnaise without sweetener or additives
1 piece whole-grain bread
Raw chicken thigh
Ketchup
1 boiled egg
1 slice carrot, boiled
2 edamame beans, shelled
5 blueberries
1 strawberry

Instructions:

1. Mix shredded cheese, diced shrimp, tomato, okra, and bell pepper with mayonnaise and lay mixture on top of a piece of whole-grain bread.

(You can substitute shrimp with tuna, chicken, or ground beef or pork and also different veggies of your choice.)

2. Heat the sandwich in a toaster oven for about 5 minutes at 320 degrees (7 minutes in a regular oven) until cheese starts to melt.
3. Stir-fry the chicken thigh with a light ketchup coating.
4. Smash the boiled egg with a fork and mix with mayo (no added salt!). Put it into a small compartment of a bento box.
5. Using a heart-shaped mold or your imagination and a knife, cut a beak out of the carrot and place it on the smashed boiled egg. Place edamame beans on the smashed egg for the bird's eyes.
6. Place blueberries, a strawberry cut in two pieces, and all the rest into your bento box.

BENTO BOXES CAN HELP YOU COMMUNICATE WITH YOUR KIDS

Bento boxes are not only a great source for a nutritional and well-balanced meal but also a great source for fun. It's easy to get a little creative when putting your child's bento box together. When your child opens his bento box at school, seeing a favorite food or funny creation can bring a smile to his face and turn his day around.

As a parent of a school-aged child, you'll probably know when a big test or competition is coming up (unless you have one of those tweens or teens who don't like to talk about school). If you know your kid has a tough science test after lunch, adding a favorite food to the bento box can help them feel more positive and ready to take the test. Or, when your kid has a game or long practice after school, you could add a large rice ball to their bento box for the extra boost of energy they'll need to do great. The point is to add foods to the bento box that can either improve their mood, improve their energy, or simply improve their day. It's easy to make food fun!

Motoko plays the "rice ball game" with her son. She'll put something inside the rice ball, like sour plum, tuna, or some small fish that her son can't tell what is inside until he takes a bite. He has fun guessing what is inside the rice ball before he eats it. This is a fun way for Motoko and her son to communicate even while apart.

And if you're really talented, you could follow the Japanese trend of making a character bento called a *Kyaraben* to brighten your child's day. From Pokémon to Winnie the Pooh to panda bears and holiday characters,

Kyarabens are a fun way to show off your skills and make your child excited to eat their food. This trend has become so popular in Japan that there are now competitions to see who can make the best-looking *Kyaraben.* Making a character bento is actually easier than it may sound. Plus, you won't be entering any competition, you'll just be making your kid happy! A quick internet search of "character bento" will surely inspire you to try your hand at making a creation of your very own.

Even though teenagers like to think they're adults, *Kyarabens* can even be made for high school students and used to increase communication between parent and child. This reminds us of a popular story in Japan. It's called "Bento Harassment" and it involves a single mother of a rebellious teenage daughter who basically stopped talking to her mom by the time she was in high school (figure 3.5). The mom starts making *Kyarabens* for her daughter to take to school. She even makes a fantastic bento box rendition of Little Red Riding Hood in which the mother's mouth is extra-large to help her better nag her daughter! Of course, this annoys the teenage girl at first, but eventually she starts to enjoy her character bento boxes. In this story, the *Kyarabens* sent to school become a tool of communication between the mother and daughter and end up strengthening their relationship. So, you see, you really can use food to communicate and improve relationships even with teenagers!

***

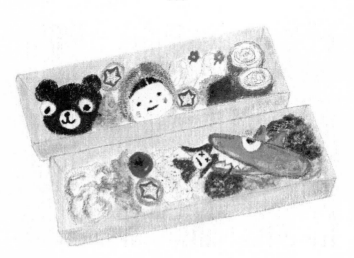

Figure 3.5   Bento Harrassment

With developing minds, hearts, and tummies, kids have a natural tendency toward novelty and excitement. Toys for kids come in every form imaginable. And that's why toys, children's clothing, children's books, and so forth, tend to be so vibrant and colorful. This is why making lunch fun to eat is the best way to go!

Shokuiku capitalizes on this feature of children, with a focus on presenting food in aesthetically vibrant, colorful, and exciting ways. From this approach, food is not simply something to be gulped down in between meetings. Rather, from this angle, food is something to be cherished, appreciated, and celebrated. Every bento box, filled with a variety of healthy food options, is screaming to bring joy and wonder to anyone who is willing to take the time to appreciate all that it includes. With its focus on food appreciation, *Shokuiku* is capitalizing on childlike wonder when it comes to the entire eating experience.

Chapter 4

Eliminating Picky Eater Syndrome

Many parents struggle with children who are picky eaters. Having a picky eater can be frustrating at times. It can also be worrying, as parents might wonder if their child is getting in the right nutrition when she insists on only ever eating a few specific foods.

Because Motoko has raised her son the *Shokuiku* way, he is an adventurous and excellent eater. But you could describe one of his friends as the complete opposite. Motoko's son has a friend who is also six years old and is an extremely picky eater who will only eat pizza and French fries. If this sounds like an exaggeration, it's not! Motoko has witnessed this multiple times when having her son's friend over to the house to eat or when dining out with the friend and his mother. On all occasions, the young boy will *insist* on only eating pizza or French fries. In fact, when he and his mother come over to Motoko's house for a meal, his mother brings ingredients to make a pizza for her picky son. When they dine out, Motoko's son will make kind recommendations of foods that he likes on the menu, to which his friend replies, "No, I only eat pizza and French fries!"

Motoko has spoken to the friend's mom about her son's picky eating habits, and, of course, she is a concerned mother. However, she is also a picky eater, often ordering pizza and French fries alongside her son. Both mother and son refuse seafood, and in one instance he refused to eat dinner at Motoko's house after smelling seafood, exclaiming, "It smells like fish—I can't eat here!" As much as the friend's mother does try to get her own son to eat more foods, Motoko has seen her quickly give up and give in to her son's demands. This situation is common in many households, but not Motoko's because, as the knowledgeable parent, she makes the final decision in what her son eats. Every time!

Does this situation sound familiar at all? If you're a typical American parent, you may have given up on some aspects of getting your kids to eat more healthy foods. With so many treats and processed foods on the market, it's getting harder and harder for parents to control the eating habits of their kids. After all, so many kids these days have developed a strong preference for processed foods early on in life. It can feel easier to just resign yourself to it. Besides, there's no denying that it's easier for you to make lunches when you're just throwing bags of premade food into the lunch box or throwing a frozen meal into the oven—set it and forget it style.

But think about this: Have you ever seen someone who grew up in an Asian country be picky about what they eat? Not as much, because of being raised with *Shokuiku* principles.

TASTE PREFERENCES IN CHILD DEVELOPMENT

When it comes to food for our kids, we need to understand the biology of food preferences across development. In short, there is often a good reason why young kids don't initially like asparagus and broccoli!

An extraordinary amount of energy is needed to help with brain development for babies and young children. The human brain is by far the most complex organ of the body, and it requires extra energy in the form of calories to develop appropriately. The foods and flavors that infants and young children prefer reinforces what we know about brain development at that age.[1]

Infants and young children have a strong preference for sweet flavors. Which is great, because breastmilk and formula are sweet and contain most of the energy young, developing brains need in the first several months of life. On the flip side, children are famously often averse to bitter flavors, like those found in many vegetables. This point seems to be rooted in the fact that many bitter vegetables actually carry low levels of toxins.[2] These toxins are benign for mature digestive systems, but they are not necessarily benign for developing digestive systems. In fact, this seems to be a primary reason why so many women across the globe tend to be averse to bitter vegetables during pregnancy.[3]

Given all these biological factors, feeding our kids healthy diets can feel like an upstream battle. That said, it is a battle that you really cannot afford to lose. And it is possible to achieve with *Shokuiku*.

SHOKUIKU PRINCIPLE: MODEL WHAT YOU WANT YOUR CHILD TO EAT

Importantly, there's no such thing as a born taste "dislike." Think about kids all over the world, who, as part of their normal diets, eat anything from stink bugs (Africa) to fried spider (Cambodia) to Spam (United States— what the heck *is* in Spam, anyway?). **We parents are the ones who teach our children to like or not like foods.**[4]

Through your own eating behavior, and your interactions with your child while they eat, you become a role model for your child—you become your child's food educator, in the same way your child mimics how you talk, words to say, and beliefs to have. If you pinch your nose and say "Ew, gross!" when offered a food you don't love, your child will develop an instinct to avoid that food as well, as though it would be actually dangerous to eat the food their parents are freaking out about. **Be aware of your own behavior with your food preferences so they don't get passed down to your children.**

In short, if you want your child to eat more fruits and vegetables but you never eat them yourself, you can bet they won't either, especially if you have a strong reaction to these foods. Instead, work on exploring new fruits and vegetables (and other healthy foods) together! *Shokuiku* has taught Marie, Motoko, and everyone else who follows it that healthy foods don't have to be boring foods. In fact, they're not boring at all—they're delicious! If you don't want your kids to be picky eaters, you can't be one either.

SHOKUIKU PRINCIPLE: VARIETY IS THE SPICE OF LIFE

The number of different flavors kids are offered is another primary factor that influences what a child's eating behavior and preferences will be.[5] A study has shown that even rats exposed to a diverse menu from birth were more apt to try new flavors later in life. From the study: "Rats who have been exposed at an early age to a variety of flavors in their diet are likelier later in life to ingest a new flavor . . . than rats reared on a more restricted diet; but this effect is not found in rats whose experience is broadened only in adulthood."[6]

Rats actually provide a great model for human food preferences, as they are omnivorous in very much the same ways humans are. It's not a coincidence that rats are found in areas that have been settled by humans all across the globe. Looking to other cultures like Japan, as well as other relevant species (e.g., rats), can shed enormous light on ways to understand and improve our diets as well as the diets of our children.

Studies have also shown that when you introduce "a variety of flavors and foods in the first two years of life, (it) may lead to acceptance of a wider variety of flavors and foods in later childhood, and may increase the likelihood of children's trying of new foods."[7]

As a nutritionist, Marie has experienced and learned about many picky eaters. From this she has found that parents who reintroduce rejected foods over and over again tend to eventually find their child accepting a once-hated food. For example, one mom she learned about was hoping to get her child to eat tomatoes. So, she kept putting tomatoes out on the table every day for about a month. And wouldn't you know it, after about a month's time the kid ate and enjoyed tomatoes! There are many other examples of kids (and adults) eventually coming around to new flavors and a wider variety of foods after being exposed to them repeatedly. Once they are familiar with the flavor, they tend to end up liking it. Experiencing varieties of tastes and learning from those tastes while children are still young will ensure they grow up being familiar with and accepting of a full palate of flavors and textures.

SHOKUIKU PRINCIPLE: *SANKAKU* (TRIANGLE) EATING

In Japan, in order to get our kids used to eating many different flavors and textures, we make sure to present food to young children—in school and at home—in a *Sankaku*, or "Triangle," method.

Instead of having a big plate in front of you with just one food like pizza or pasta, in Japan we prepare three to five smaller plates with different foods and arrange them in a loose triangle in front of the child (figure 4.1). Importantly, the parent decides the portion appropriate for the child, rather than the child piling up only the foods they want in too large of quantities.

You see, when eating from just one big plate, you constantly eat with no pause. Food is gulped down, and American parents tend to sometimes "force" children to eat everything on the plate. While we also don't like wasting food in Japan, we serve only what a child can eat (and they can always ask for more).

Even more detrimental, because in America meals are often loaded with significantly more than a person of that age and size needs and is largely

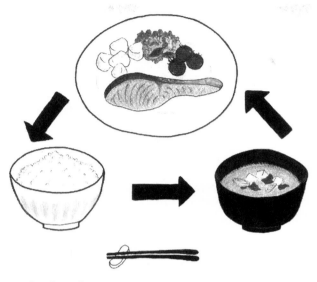

Figure 4.1 Triangle eating

processed or unhealthy, this is leading to not only picky eating syndrome but also a slew of health problems we'll cover in a later chapter.

With the Triangle eating method, a child takes a bite from each plate evenly one-by-one until they eat every kind of food. Then, they go back to repeat the pattern, until they finish everything. This way, a child can eat a variety of foods evenly at one mealtime. Kids can pause every time they carry food to their mouths, so there's plenty of time to chew and taste and enjoy each food. This way, they're eating fairly slowly, letting them realize they don't have to eat too much to be full. This helps them regulate listening to their bodies so they aren't overeating in the future.

We introduce a new ingredient every week, and we increase the number of ingredients to approximately 30 a day to make sure there is significant variety in what our kids are eating. We also try to serve varying lunches and dinners every day, so we are not eating the same thing every day all week. Japanese school lunches don't repeat a lunch for an entire month! Now, we know that sounds like a big challenge, and you don't have to go to that extreme, but the more you do this, the less picky your child will be.

It's easy to do Triangle eating at home, since you're probably presenting all foods at the same time during meals. But it can be a challenge to have your kids eat in this way at restaurants. In countries like the United States, France, and Italy, waiters tend to bring one course out at a time. You're probably used to getting an appetizer first, followed by a salad or soup, then the main dish, all separated by an amount of time probably determined by your waiter. And while the waiter is doing this because it is customary in these countries, you can easily ask him or her to bring out all the dishes at the same time. That's what Motoko does while out with her son. She asks the waiter to bring all her son's food out at once so he can eat using the Triangle method. This allows Motoko's son to eat all meals in a consistent way and continue to try new foods.

You can even practice Triangle eating when out at an Italian restaurant where free bread is often brought to the table almost immediately. Motoko is always terrified when the bread basket is dropped off! She's worried her son will ruin his appetite by eating the seemingly continuous free supply of bread that her son, of course, loves. What she does (and you can too) is have her son eat and enjoy one piece of the yummy bread and ask the waiter to bring her son's order out soon after. Problem solved!

To eliminate picky eating, kids need to try one certain food many times before getting used to the taste and starting to like it. It's important to let them eat a variety of foods at one meal and keep doing that until picky eating habits disappear. Kids can also challenge themselves when eating foods they're not fond of by checking how much food is left on each plate for them to finish up.

The triangle of food should change from day to day. When it comes to appealing to the curious, adventurous minds of children, this is a good thing!

If you, as a parent, don't like the food that's on a plate, try eating with your kids and challenge yourself so you can also try to enjoy the wonderful taste of real foods that you haven't explored before. Kids are watching you. If you can be a good example, kids will be sure to follow. And why not use this opportunity to create healthier eating habits for yourself and extend your life as well?

And if you think you will throw up if you eat something you hate and can't hide it? You can be honest about it, tell your child you wish your parents had been able to offer you that food so that you could enjoy it, and try it again together. Say, "I want to broaden my world and try this with you!" More exposure to the food you've hated may also help *you* develop a new taste!

SHOKUIKU PRINCIPLE: DON'T HIDE FLAVORS

In Japan, we identify five taste profiles. **Salty** foods have minerals inside for health. **Umami** is a taste found in foods like seaweed or broth that contain amino acids. Kids may have an aversion to **bitter** and **sour** foods initially because they may taste as though they've spoiled to young palates. And **sweet** foods give us energy.

In America, it's a popular strategy to hide vegetables in food to get kids to eat them. There are entire cookbooks that teach parents how to sneak healthy foods into children's diets. This never has to be done in Japan. You shouldn't have to go to such lengths! The vegetables and healthy foods you serve your child should be spotlighted and celebrated. Your child is so lucky to be served something so fresh and healthy! You need to shift your thinking from "This is something I *have* to get my child to eat" to "This is a food my child *gets* to eat, and let's praise the flavor and benefits."

For babies and toddlers, *never* hide the original taste of the food by adding unnecessary sweetness or saltiness. The youngest tots should experience the original taste of whole foods as they are. This means avoiding the use of sugar or any other sweeteners, salt, or condiments that drastically change the true flavor of foods, especially for babies and toddlers. Kids need to learn the original taste of the whole foods. This will help them continue to explore and enjoy more of the foods they have never encountered before. Above all, when kids grow up avoiding (or at least limiting) the taste of sweetness and saltiness, it helps them bypass those foods in the future, therefore lowering their chances of future obesity and certain lifestyle-related diseases.

As children get older and start preschool and elementary school, you can start adding light seasonings like salt and other spices to accentuate flavors. But do your best to use the minimum, and still avoid sugar!

SHOKUIKU PRINCIPLE: HARVEST TOGETHER

Deep-rooted cultural traditions regarding food underscore the beauty and importance of natural foods. Japanese culture, which surrounds all the ideas of *Shokuiku*, offers a significant counterexample to the food culture of the United States based on the principles of *Shokuiku*, where the origins of food is a critical part of the experience of eating. When children are taught to understand where their food comes from, they develop a self-aware approach to eating. Further, such an enlightened approach to eating leads to a deep appreciation for many natural foods, which are, proportionately, much more common in Japanese cuisine than in American cuisine.

To help spotlight the glory of natural foods rather than hiding them, all Japanese children take a school trip every year called *Imo-hori*. The

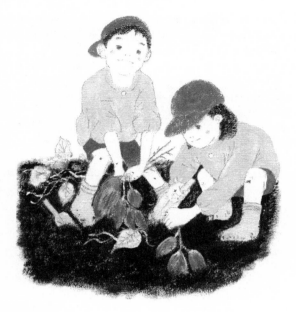

Figure 4.2 IMOHORI

word *Imo-hori* roughly translates to "digging for sweet potatoes." And the day entails exactly that (figure 4.2). This is mostly a day for kindergarteners in Japan, but older kids often help the younger ones pull the sweet potatoes from the earth. Once the harvest is over, the children partake in *Yakiimo*, or baking the sweet potatoes they've just pulled themselves. The day is full of conversation, learning, and bonding among the young students. It's a great way for the children of Japan to feel interconnected, since it's a tradition for all. The children even get to take any leftover harvested sweet potatoes home. When they do this, the kids get to tell their family all about their fun day of digging for sweet potatoes and talk about what they learned.

So to mimic this, take *your* child to the nearest farmers' market or farm. Include them in the purchase of the foods you are trying to sneak into their dinner. Show them their vibrant colors. Let them hear the conversation you have with the farmer about how they're grown. Find out why a certain fruit tastes sweet—perhaps it was grown in a tropical area. You don't need to know everything about how a food is grown, but your child can be part of those conversations.

Better yet, let them grow a small garden with you, even on the patio, to see the magic of a food going from seed to a beautiful, edible plant. Let them pick it from the ground and wash it. They are so much more likely to not balk at eating a food when they know where it comes from and why they're eating it. For example, many American kids hate tomatoes. But if you grow beautiful tomatoes in your backyard and the kids are part of the process, learning how long it takes and all the steps needed, they will start believing that the tomato is precious. At the farmers' market, encourage them to thank the farmer in person as well—it fosters a lifelong appreciation for the foods that truly feed our bodies.

Consider grapes compared to Oreos, as an example. In the United States, if you're throwing a party for a bunch of eight-year-olds and you put out some snacks, it's common to offer various processed options—think Oreos—as well as (often based on mom-guilt) various non-processed options, such as grapes. Any American parent will tell you that the Oreos will usually be long gone before the grapes are barely touched in such a scenario. But if kids had a better understanding of where these two different food options come from, they might think twice. Grapes are grown on hillsides in regions around the world that are surrounded by natural beauty. They are carefully attended to by farmers and they are, quite literally, sun-kissed. Oreos, on the other hand, are made of a dizzying array of human-made chemicals. (Fun fact about Oreos: They are actually vegan friendly. This is not because they have much in the way of vegetables in them. Rather, it's because human-made chemicals take the place of anything that might remotely pass for an animal product.)

Shokuiku provides a system for getting children to truly understand where their food comes from. And this understanding plays a role in catalyzing healthy eating habits that include a wide variety of foods.

In addition to a focus on food origins, *Shokuiku* has a clear focus on food appreciation. This tradition has the capacity to make children mindful about food, discouraging kids from taking their food for granted. Food is always something to be thankful for—especially considering the fact that human history is filled with stories of famine and starvation. Regular reminders that food is a gift has the capacity to build in true appreciation for food—an attribute that will pay dividends across your child's entire life span.

SHOKUIKU PRINCIPLE: DON'T GIVE UP

You might be disappointed and frustrated to see your baby spitting out what you've made for him or her, but you need to tell yourself that every rejection is not a failure—it is an important taste experience for your baby. By eating different kinds of food, little by little, they expand their world of taste.

Don't take a rejection of food as permanent or as a failure on what you prepared. Every food just takes getting used to, and with repetitive exposure your child will develop an expansive taste acceptance. It's not that in Japan children never say no to a food at first. It's just that in Japan we don't give up on serving it. Research shows that a child needs to be introduced to a food up to 15 times before he or she will accept it.[8] And another study shows that new foods may need to be offered to preschool-aged children 10 to 16 times before acceptance occurs.[9]

For example, a food's bitterness or sourness may be naturally avoided because bitterness can be interpreted as poisonous and sourness as spoiled. So, when we introduce those types of foods, kids first don't want to eat them. Parents tend to think if they skip those foods when children are young, their child will naturally appreciate those types of foods when they're older. But it doesn't often work that way. People learn to get used to a taste as they eat the same food over and over, little by little. This means it is important for you to let your kids eat as many different types of foods as many times as possible for them to start liking the tastes. It has been scientifically proven that the "introduction of a variety of flavors and foods in the first two years of life may lead to acceptance of a wider variety of flavors and foods in later childhood and may increase the likelihood of children's trying of new foods."[10]

SO, HOW DO I GET MY KID TO TRY NEW FOODS?

As we've said (and as you may know), it can be extremely frustrating to prepare food for your child and have them spit it out, throw it off their high-chair, or block the spoon from their mouth. To counter act this, **be excited about the foods you're giving your child, and eat them too.** Motoko will enthusiastically say, "Wow, this food came from the ocean!" Or, "Do you hear how the cucumber and celery clicks and snaps when we bite it?" Just like making kids put on their shoes or do chores like cleaning up, making food fun can mean more success at the dinner table. Remember how your parents used to pretend an airplane or train was delivering a spoon into baby's mouth? It works!

If you're eating something with a little more spice and your child wants to try it, let them! Let your child know what it might taste like, then offer a small amount. Whether they like it or not is not the point. The point is that it builds trust and connection through eating with you. Applaud them for trying it and encourage their adventurous attitude about eating! This will also help with reducing picky eating if children see you enjoying lots of foods.

Another tip to decreasing mealtime fights is making sure your child is active enough during the day. Too many American parents (and parents in general) allow their children to be extremely sedate all day. The more active a child is, the hungrier they'll be, and the less you'll hear them fighting over what they're offered to eat. Hungry children make for less picky children. This is a great opportunity to talk about how the food they're eating makes them have all the energy they need to do their activities.

Having meals with people outside your immediate family can also be beneficial. Take advantage of an opportunity to eat with different friends and family members once in a while and experience the cuisine and preparations of food they enjoy. This will help broaden your child's taste horizons. Talk with your kids about why a family member or friend eats a particular food or dish and use the conversation to teach about other cultures. This makes eating exciting! Kids are naturally curious, and if they see their friends or others eating a food they were refusing before, it will help them want to try it without any force at all.

WHAT ABOUT SUPPLEMENTS FOR NUTRITION?

Americans sometimes rely on supplements to try to conveniently bypass the beneficial foods they should be eating. And while supplements can certainly fill a void sometimes, they will never replace the real thing. It's impossible to perfectly replicate nature and the way our digestive system works with real food. Your body won't digest and absorb the nutrients from supplements as efficiently as it will from fresh, whole foods. Just think, supplements are a relatively new invention, but food has been around forever!

Unfortunately, many supplements have more than just vitamins and minerals in them. Many tout high percentanges of the nutrients your body needs, but they are also, sometimes, chock-full of sugar, heavily processed, or not properly balanced. And don't forget the fact that supplements aren't regulated, which means they can contain ingredients that aren't even on their label.

***

People have evolved to prefer sweet foods that can lead to fat storage if eaten in excess. But we have also evolved to desire a broader range of foods. Our ancestors lived off diets that were fully based on natural foods. *Shokuiku* capitalizes on these features of our evolved food psychology by underscoring the beauty of both natural foods and food variety. Using the *Shokuiku* methods for teaching kids about food has the capacity to encourage preferences for a wide variety of natural, whole foods. And when cultivated carefully and mindfully, these food preferences have the capacity to have all kinds of physical, emotional, and social benefits across one's life span.

With its focus on natural foods, food variety, and playful, aesthetic presentation, *Shokuiku* harnesses child psychology related to food in a way that cultivates an appreciation for more healthful foods. This approach discourages picky eating in a systemic way, getting kids to appreciate and even get excited about new kinds of foods.

Do you want your kid to gravitate toward healthy, whole food options? And be open to novel cuisines and types of foods? *Shokuiku* is the answer.

Food isn't only about eating—it's about learning and enjoying the world! With *Shokuiku*, your child will grow up to be able to enjoy foods from any culture and location. If you grow up being a picky eater and can't, or won't, eat fish for example, how can you enjoy the gorgeous culture of sushi? **As parents, not providing *Shokuiku* means depriving your child of a major joy in life!**

Chapter 5

Improving Children's Behavior

You've just read about *Shokuiku* during that precious baby stage, but there is still much to learn! There are so many things you can do to improve your child's health and even their behavior through nutrition. That's right, *Shokuiku* is not just for babies. It can be used for toddlers, school-aged children, moody teenagers, and even adults. In this chapter, you'll learn more about *Shokuiku* during the toddler and school years, and Marie and Motoko will share personal stories of how they've seen food help children's behaviors with their own eyes.

Being a parent to young children (especially toddlers) could be described as a fun and exhausting adventure. The exhaustion comes from many places, like constantly chasing your children and trying to get them to listen to you. How many times do you have to ask your child to put on shoes before leaving the house before he finally does so? Or how often does your child actually brush her teeth after the first time you tell her to? All young children have completely normal moments of hyperactivity and not listening to their parents (or is it selective listening?). But what if you start to notice your child is having a hard time sitting still and concentrating almost constantly? Or what if your child sometimes results to anger and aggression after something doesn't go his way? If these scenarios sound familiar, you are not alone!

As a nutritionist, Motoko's mother had seen hundreds of parents struggling with every behavioral issue a child can have. She saw plenty of kids dealing with aggression, poor concentration, and hyperactivity. Did you know some of these behaviors can be linked to food? As an example, a high intake of sugar for breakfast can make your child hyperactive and hard to control before his inevitable crash. But just like some foods can cause poor behavior in children, other foods can help improve behavior. **This means the foods you provide your school-aged child can have a major positive impact on her ability to learn and retain information while in class,** *as long as these foods are nutrient-dense and not calorie-dense.*

But breakfast is not the only meal that impacts your child's behavior. All meals and snacks are important. The ultimate test of how food can improve aggressive behavior happened when Oxford University gave supplements made up of vitamins, minerals, and fatty acids to prison inmates and found that doing so led to 26% less antisocial and aggressive behavior with at least two weeks of supplementation.[1] If nutrition can help adult criminals in just two weeks, think of what it can do for your developing child!

JAPANESE SCHOOL LUNCHES (*KYUSHOKU*) AND THE *SHOKUIKU* BASIC LAW

In Japan, government officials noticed with the burgeoning invasion of Western food establishments and culture such as fast-food chains and convenience stores selling candy, that the population—youths especially—became more obese and less attentive at school. So, they enacted a *Shokuiku* (food education) Basic Law in 2005.[2] With this law, thousands of school nutritionists were hired and children were *required* to eat the school's catered lunch to help kids' behaviors (figure 5.1). Formulated to promote healthier dietary habits from a young age, lunchtime at school for Japanese kids became a learning experience versus just a break between classes.

Kyushoku (or school lunches) in Japan differ greatly from the fairly chaotic and noisy cafeterias Americans are used to seeing. During *Kyushoku*, the students are greatly involved in the preparation and cleanup of the healthy foods chosen by each school's nutritionist. Marie, a nutritionist herself, says there are three purposes of *Kyushoku*: to keep students healthy by providing them with nutritious foods, to let students experience and explore Japanese food culture using local seasonal ingredients, and to teach students to greatly appreciate the people who are involved in making their lunches, including farmers, kitchen staff, and anyone who helps to prepare the meals.

During *Kyushoku*:

- First- to sixth-grade students help to dish out school lunches while wearing special uniforms and masks (figure 5.2). This lets the children be a part of preparing their own food they are about to eat and helps them learn to appreciate the meal that has been cooked for them by others.

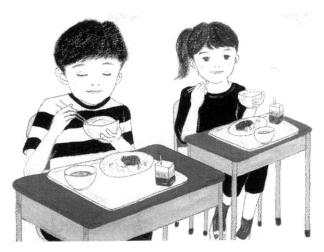

Figure 5.1   School Lunch

- Once they are done eating, the students clean the classroom where they ate their lunch with brooms and towels, leaving no food left on desks and floors for the rest of the school day. With full bellies and a clean classroom, they can quickly get back to learning!

Every school in Japan has a nutritionist who plans the students' lunch menu a month in advance, and this ensures the students will eat a variety of nutritious foods. The nutritionists put great thought into the menu and always make sure to use seasonal vegetables. They also consider festive dishes for the students to enjoy. It's also the job of the nutritionists to make sure each meal meets the targeted nutritional value. That's a lot of work!

Students in Japan won't see the same *Kyushoku* menu within the same month. This means the students are fortunate to experience a wide variety of foods and flavors, which helps them expand their palates and acceptance of many foods. These hard-working Japanese nutritionists plan lunch dishes in a way that the students don't have to eat the same things over and over again. This means the same type of protein wouldn't be served for many days in a row, which could look like fish on Monday, pork on Tuesday, soy on Wednesday, beef on Thursday, and chicken on Friday. Japanese children even get to experience foods from different cultures during lunchtime. American students would be so fortunate to have their school nutritionists

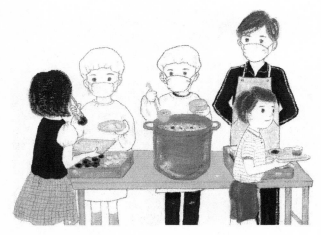

Figure 5.2   School Lunch 2

plan their lunches in this way. As a matter of fact, American students would be fortunate just to have a school nutritionist on staff!

As part of the *Shokuiku* Basic Law, Japanese students are also taught where the food they eat comes from, and why it helps their bodies. They are presented food using the Triangle method (discussed in chapter 4), and they can't leave the table until they finish their meal. Kids of all nations tend to want to do the same things as their peers, so when all the students are eating the same thing, acceptance of the food goes up. But if a child refuses to eat, they have to sit there until they comply, for hours if that's what it takes. (Fortunately, school lunches in Japan are well-portioned, so the students that must stay and eat won't be stuffing themselves like a Thanksgiving turkey!) This may sound authoritarian or cruel, but it causes students in Japan to try new foods, which helps eliminate picky eating habits.

At first glance, *Kyushoku* sounds like an impossible thing to do in America. And maybe that's true to a certain degree. It's hard to envision American schools enacting anything like *Kyushoku*, isn't it? But that doesn't mean you can't adopt some of these ideas and implement them in your home. One of the simplest ideas when feeding your children is to give them a variety of foods to try from a young age, like the way children in Japan get to try new foods at school. This variety will help your children eventually grow to enjoy many foods besides chicken nuggets and cheese pizza and not have so many foods they dislike (or think they dislike) even when they're adults. Food can be a wonderful adventure, and the best way to experience food is to try it all!

Kyushoku vs. American School Lunch

As you can imagine, *Kyushoku* is very different from an American school lunch in many ways. While there is something in America called the National School Lunch Program (NSLP) from the USDA, this program is optional and not mandated. Schools must meet certain standards to enact the NSLP, but they get government reimbursements if they do so.[3] Students in America can get these meals for free or for a reduced price if their family is eligible based on income. There are standards for serving sizes and types of foods served as a part of the NSLP, and these include requirements for food groups like fruits, vegetables, grains, meats, and milk.[4]

While these efforts from the USDA have definitely improved school lunches in America, the problem of school-aged kids not consuming the right types of foods to fuel their bodies and brains during lunch (and breakfast) remains. For instance, not 100% of children in school are participating in the NSLP, with many bringing lunch from home and/or buying extra snacks and treats from the cafeteria or school vending machines (side note—Japanese schools don't even have vending machines!). American children also get more food options at lunch compared to Japanese children, and this freedom can often lead to an unbalanced meal full of processed snacks and treats. Also, unlike Japanese children participating in *Kyushoku*, American schoolchildren are never made to try new foods or finish their entire meals before returning to class. They also never take turns serving the food and cleaning up after their classmates like their Japanese peers do.

In Japan, students don't have designated snack times or even try to sneak snacks during classes (except for maybe the very small children who need a little something in their tummies more often). Their only food while at school is lunch. But since Japanese students eat a well-balanced and nourishing breakfast in the morning, they're hungry but not *too* hungry by the time lunch rolls around. Their level of hunger at lunch encourages Japanese students to *want* to eat their entire nutritious lunch. They actually find the foods to be tastier when they are hungry. Hunger is the best seasoning, after all!

American students who skip breakfast or snack all day long at school may be less likely to eat their entire healthy lunch their parents packed for them. If snacks are suggested at your child's school, try choosing something that will be good for their digestion once lunchtime hits. A nice piece of fruit, like an apple or banana, would be a perfect choice for giving your kid a little extra energy until lunchtime while not being too filling to turn them away from their midday meal.

These differences leave American children at a disadvantage and with much less knowledge about nutrition, trying new foods, and respecting the food and people who made it. Although you as a parent can't change the rules and regulations of American school cafeterias, you can change what your child eats for lunch each day. Remember the fun and tasty bento boxes you learned to make in chapter 3? These could really come in handy for school lunches! By sending your child to school with a bento box made of one-third protein, one-third carbs, and one-third veggies you can help them refuel properly and have the brain power and proper energy to finish their school day in a positive way. You'll soon read about how the types of foods kids eat before and during school have a major impact on their day, with some foods fueling school performance and others fueling bad behavior and poor learning.

HOW BREAKFAST AFFECTS BEHAVIOR AT SCHOOL

Making sure your child starts their day off right with a nourishing breakfast before going to school is super important, and we know from research that kids who never skip breakfast tend to have better academic performance and behavior in school than breakfast skippers.[5] Many studies have shown that kids who start their day with a healthy breakfast have more energy, better concentration, higher grades, normal body weights, better behavior, and even overall better diets than their peers who skip breakfast or eat one that is high in calories and sugar and low in nutrition.[6]

The word *breakfast* literally means "break the fast." Your body slows down while you sleep, leading to decreased blood sugar, a state of fasting by the time you wake up, and low energy. That's why parents need coffee in the morning! If children skip breakfast before heading off to school, they may be met with poor concentration, crankiness, sleepiness, and a lack of motivation, all factors that certainly won't help your kid learn, grow, and develop. Not to mention that by the time kids who skip breakfast get to lunch, they may feel so ravenously hungry that they'll eat anything in sight (but not the veggies). When kids show up to lunch this hungry, all hope of eating a healthy lunch goes out the window due to strong cravings for extra snacks and sweets available in the cafeteria or from a nearby friend.

Besides simply eating breakfast, the glycemic load of a child's morning meal is another important determinate of how well the school day will go.

Research has shown that children who eat a high-glycemic breakfast, or one that is high in sugar, display more negative behaviors like frustration, poor concentration, and poor performance when compared to children who eat a low-glycemic breakfast.[7] When a low-glycemic (low-sugar) breakfast is eaten by children, they not only demonstrate better memory, information retention, and focus, but get less frustrated than their higher-sugar-breakfast peers.[8]

After Motoko moved to the United States and enrolled her son in school, she received a surprising email that was sent to her and the rest of the parents at her son's new school. The email was about breakfast and was sent by school directors with the hope of influencing parents to feed their kids a healthier breakfast before sending them to school. The school asked the parents to stop feeding their children sugary cereals and other high-sugar breakfast foods in the morning. They also wanted to make sure the students were not skipping breakfast on school days.

The email went on to say that teachers and other authority figures at the school could fully tell which children skipped breakfast, which children had a high-sugar breakfast, and which children ate a well-balanced, nutritious breakfast. They could tell because the breakfast skippers were very tired until they ate lunch and the high-sugar breakfast eaters were arriving at school in very active and hyper moods but would eventually crash once class began. Motoko was shocked! In Japan, she had never heard of kids skipping breakfast or eating a high-sugar breakfast. This was all news to her!

This story goes to show that the simple act of eating breakfast is not enough to improve your child's behavior and test scores in school. His breakfast must be one that contains plenty of nutrition and healthy calories that will keep his energy and brain power up all day, or at least until lunchtime. As if the behavioral benefits weren't enough, eating a well-balanced breakfast can also improve your child's overall health, including their digestive health, metabolism, bone health, and heart health. Kids who eat breakfast regularly have also been shown to have an easier time maintaining their body weight than breakfast skippers, and we all know how difficult *that* can be as adults!

BRIBING KIDS TO GO TO SCHOOL WITH SUGAR

More times than she can count, Motoko has witnessed children being bribed to go to school with candy and other sweets for breakfast by their well-intentioned parents (figure 5.3). What tends to happen is these candy-eating children end up acting restless and hyper in class due to the sugar high induced from eating candy and sweets on an empty stomach. Then comes the inevitable crash that occurs once these kids' blood sugars plummet after the intense blood sugar spike that was the result of their supersweet breakfast. But the parents don't see the crash because that takes place once their child is settled in the classroom. Parents only see a child that is awake, alert, and ready for the day when they drop them off in the carpool lane. The teachers are then left with a zonked-out kid who is coming down from a sugar high. Lucky teachers!

Of course, as all parents know, sometimes bribery is completely necessary, so we're definitely not trying to shame anyone here! Sometimes you really need just a few minutes of silence, and a cookie is the only way to get that. **The simple truth is that sugary cereals and donuts are not the best breakfast options for fuel and that these types of breakfasts cause kids to be hyper in class and then crash, leading to a disruption in their ability to learn.** Parents need to know that sugar intake, and especially sugar intake on an empty stomach before school, has consequences.

Whether you have been feeding your child sugar for breakfast or have bribed your child with treats before school, we as parents are all just trying to do our best. No one ever said parenting was easy! But now that you

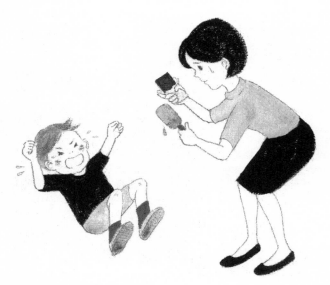

Figure 5.3   Bribing a kid with sweets

have been armed with more information about what happens when kids eat a high-sugar breakfast before school, you can make the needed changes to ensure they are behaving and learning properly. Children really do want to go to school and learn, and oftentimes a child will eventually choose to go to school on their own without the enticing bribery of sugar. We promise!

HOW AN EATING SCHEDULE CAN HELP

Another aspect of *Shokuiku* that can help improve your child's behavior at school and at home is to implement an eating schedule. But an eating schedule can be beneficial for the entire family.

Life in America tends to be so busy that meals are rushed through or skipped altogether. How many times have you rushed out the door in the morning with nothing in you but a cup of coffee (if you're lucky)? One of the beautiful things about *Shokuiku* is that it encourages you to take a moment to honor and reflect on the food you are about to eat before your meal and be thankful for the meal afterwards (more on this in the next chapter). Eating in this reflective and mindful manner also leads to slower-paced and more enjoyable mealtimes, especially when these meals are shared with others. Plus, you become more aware of when you're truly hungry and when you're satisfied and ready to stop eating without getting overly full.

When you have a good understanding of proper nutrition and know that eating a variety of foods can lead to improved health and more longevity, you and your family will stop skipping meals. **And when you take even just a moment to think about what you are about to put into your body, you may be surprised to see your food choices evolve from calorie-dense to nutrient-dense.** The good news is, nutrient-dense foods (especially those that contain fiber, lean protein, and healthy fats) tend to be more filling, helping you reach satiety sooner and prevent overeating on a regular basis.

Following an eating schedule can help families stay on track with regularly eating highly nutritious (and delicious) foods. And if you can learn to be more mindful around when your body needs food, and when it has had enough food, you will probably start noticing a pattern of how often you need to eat. Although your schedule is probably different from the person next to you, at least having set windows of time that you and your family eat meals and snacks can be helpful. Many people feel their best when they eat either a meal or small snack every two to three hours during the waking hours, but this is not a hard and fast rule.

With that in mind, here is an example of an eating schedule:

7:00 a.m. Breakfast
9:30 a.m. Snack
12:30 p.m. Lunch
3:00 p.m. Snack
6:00 p.m. Dinner
8:30 p.m. Snack

This schedule is only meant to be an example and can be easily tweaked to fit the needs of your family. You may find that three snacks per day is more than you need, or that you need four healthy snacks per day to feel satisfied and energized. It's unrealistic to be able to follow an exact eating schedule every single day, just like it's unrealistic to follow a strict and restrictive diet full of food rules. The fact that *Shokuiku* does not ask you to eliminate entire food groups or only eat at certain times of the day means you have the freedom to find both the best foods and the best eating schedule that will work for your family!

DEALING WITH TODDLER FOOD BEHAVIORS AND TANTRUMS

Shokuiku teaches parents to feed their children healthy foods from day one. Parents are also taught to share an appreciation and understanding of where food comes from with their children. This type of relationship with food can stick with children well into adulthood and can even help parents avoid those "terrible twos" or toddler tantrums that often happen at the kitchen table. You probably know what we're talking about here, those intense tantrums from a picky eater where your precious toddler resorts to throwing dishes, smashing food, and even spitting.

Having a picky eater is somewhat dreaded. What is worse than taking the time and thought to prepare a well-balanced meal for your toddler only to have them *literally* throw it in your face? These food tantrums can quickly result in toddlers completely skipping their meal, eating only a few bites of what you prepared for them, or only eating less-nourishing snack foods that you finally gave into for the sake of some much-needed quiet time (for you).

There are many ways picky eating habits and food tantrums may develop in babies and toddlers, including early feeding difficulties, late introduction of solid foods, and pressure from parents to eat.[9] What can result is an overall poor variety of accepted foods that can lead to nutrient deficiencies, especially iron and zinc, two important minerals needed for normal growth and development.[10] Although some picky eating habits can be just a normal part of toddlerhood, if you have a toddler or young child whose behavior during mealtimes is causing poor health outcomes, it may be time to intervene.

So, what can you do to fix or completely skip the mealtime tantrums phase? The philosophies of *Shokuiku* can help. One of the most important things *Shokuiku* encourages is eating as a family, which promotes many positive benefits for babies and toddlers, including a higher acceptance of a wide variety of healthy foods. Oftentimes, parents can avoid raising picky eaters by simply feeding their young children the same healthy foods they eat during meals and snacks. This could include giving your baby, who has just started solid foods, small pieces of your supersoft, steamed vegetables at dinner or bites of soft fruits. And giving babies a wide variety of fresh, whole foods from the start can help develop their tastebuds for things like fruits and vegetables that you would never dream of a baby or small child enjoying. Gone are the days of needing to wait until your baby is much older to try foods like yogurt, fish, and eggs. You can give your baby much more than just rice cereal and mushed carrots! Again, you can help your baby develop a yearning for many different types of healthy foods by offering them repeatedly.

Shokuiku also teaches eating meals without distractions, like television and electronic devices. Although we'll touch on this subject more in the next chapter, it's important to mention this now as we discuss the idea of fostering appropriate mealtime behaviors in toddlers. As a parent, it's your job to create a calm environment for your toddler when necessary, and a calm environment is necessary for a calm meal. Think about it—do you feel relaxed and like you can really enjoy your meal and be mindful about what you are eating if the TV is on or the music is turned up, or while you are scrolling through social media? Probably not! And we can't expect our young children to feel relaxed in that environment either. Removing all distractions while your family sits down together for a meal can help improve everyone's relationship with food, including the youngest family members. You can set the example for how you would like your picky toddler to eat and behave during meals by eating and enjoying the same foods along with your child.

Before we move on, it's important that we remind parents that perfection is impossible, especially when it comes to food, and that's okay! It's essential for parents to do their best to remain calm during meals, especially meals that are not going well in terms of what and how much your child is eating. Becoming panicked or stressed if your baby or toddler doesn't want to eat much food will be unhelpful, and these emotions could rub off on your little one. You shouldn't be the one having the tantrum! There will be many meals when your toddler barely eats anything, but as long as they are getting a variety of foods in over the week and they are thriving, all is not lost.

SHOKUIKU AND ADHD BEHAVIORS

At the age of six, Motoko's son was diagnosed with attention-deficit/hyperactivity disorder, or ADHD, a mental disorder that affects many children, as well as adults.[11] Symptoms of ADHD can vary, but some of the more common ones include hyperactivity and trouble sitting still, inability to pay close attention to details, lack of focus and concentration, disorganization, forgetfulness, and poor follow-through.[12] While some people can have borderline ADHD, Motoko's son has a "full-blown" case.

The prevalence of ADHD diagnoses has increased by 42% in America in the last eight years, with over 6% of children carrying the diagnosis.[13] ADHD tends to occur more often in children and is a common culprit of behavioral issues that many parents want to correct for the sake of both their child and themselves. **As of 2014, 6.4 million American children had been diagnosed with ADHD, with males being almost three times more likely to be diagnosed than females; the average age of diagnosis was seven, with symptoms typically starting between ages three and six.**[14] The earliest age a person can be formally diagnosed with ADHD is six. And although Motoko was pretty sure her son had ADHD when he was younger, he went through several long tests over the course of one week before he was finally diagnosed and could start treatment.

There are many ways to treat ADHD, and what may work for one person may not work for another. Some children and adults with ADHD use medication to treat their symptoms, while others, like Motoko's son, use a combination of medication, therapy, and food for treatment. Interestingly, foods that are high in additives and refined sugars and low in essential fatty acids have been linked to ADHD reactions in children,[15] but food cannot *cause* ADHD or cure it. Proper nutrition can be used as a *complementary treatment* for this disorder, meaning that it may make a difference in a person's ADHD symptoms if used along with other measures like medication and/or treatment.

It's important to point out that people are born with ADHD. This disorder can sometimes cause issues like aggression, lack of focus, inability to control emotions, and restlessness, especially in children. These behavioral issues can especially be a problem for school-aged children with ADHD who may find themselves in the principal's office more often than parents would like.

Proper food education, or *Shokuiku*, can be one of the complementary treatments that may help improve the overall behavior and attention span of children with ADHD, and this can even be applied to babies.[16] After working with many children in her career, Motoko's mother recalls that the ones who had been properly fed were the ones with the longest attention spans. And even if your child does not have ADHD, a proper diet can be the difference between a well-behaved child and a poorly behaved child in school, even if your child is dealing with aggressive behaviors.

Foods can increase or decrease violent, aggressive behavior. Just ask science:

- Experts agree that nutrition, or lack thereof, can contribute to violent behavior. The brain doesn't function as it should when it's fed mostly processed and packaged foods, and poor nutrition can make people more irritable and angry.[17]
- Through his research, Nobel Prize–winning chemist Linus Pauling made the case for using nutrition to help treat mental diseases. Basically, Pauling believed that you could use substances like vitamins, minerals, and enzymes alongside medications and other treatments for psychiatric disorders, like ADHD.[18]
- Dietary supplements containing vitamins, minerals, and the essential fatty acids omega-6 and omega-3 may help improve antisocial behaviors.[19]

Some kids with ADHD have been found to be sensitive to certain food ingredients, including food additives and refined sugars, that cause an increase in behavioral issues.[20] Other children may have ADHD symptoms exacerbated by nutrient deficiencies, which can be brought on by a chronically poor diet. Again, a poor diet full of sugar, salt, pesticides, and food additives does not *cause* ADHD, as children are born with it. But these types of foods may be responsible for making some symptoms like hyperactivity, aggression, and poor attention span worse.

On the flip side, there is evidence that making positive dietary changes, like removing or reducing sugar intake and eating more fresh fruits and vegetables, whole grains, fish, and plant-based protein, can help reduce ADHD symptoms (yay!). These findings suggest that diet modifications can play a significant role in the management of ADHD when used alongside other treatments, like medication and behavioral therapy.[21]

Research and parents of children with ADHD can both back up claims that food can impact ADHD symptoms in both positive and negative ways. And food can be used as medicine for many health issues and mental disorders besides ADHD. **Even if you don't have ADHD, you may still be able to recall at least one time when your mood and actions were affected by food you ate.** Perhaps you ate a large amount of sugar in one sitting and found yourself feeling overly energized and jittery until you eventually crashed. Or perhaps you can remember a time when you ate a well-balanced meal of fresh vegetables, whole grains, lean protein, and healthy fats and felt satisfied and energized for the rest of the day. Food can even affect you on an emotional level, and this can start from day one, as certain foods (like those rich in magnesium or healthy fats) can help soothe a baby and, eventually, lead to sleep.[22]

Motoko's son was diagnosed with ADHD when he was six years old, but she had a feeling he would be diagnosed with the disorder before he was old enough to sit through the testing. In fact, he had trouble ever sitting still. He also found it difficult to focus on mundane tasks, was forgetful, and was showing aggressive behaviors by the time he was in school. When he was first diagnosed, Motoko initially thought medication would not be necessary to treat his symptoms. She quickly learned that it absolutely was. After doing some research and talking with doctors and therapists, Motoko decided to start her son on medication for his ADHD. He was also treated with behavioral therapy and food.

The summer after he was diagnosed with ADHD, Motoko's son attended a camp also attended by his therapists. They saw some of his aggression firsthand while at camp. But, seemingly miraculously, he had become very stable in his behavior by that fall. His therapists were surprised by the swift improvements in his ADHD symptoms and wondered what he had done different. They had never seen such quick improvements in a child's symptoms! When the therapists learned that Motoko had been treating her son with a combination of medication, therapy, and food, they felt that his healthy diet was the X factor in his improvements, especially since they noticed that his meals were healthier than many of his peers.

Motoko shared with her son's therapists that she had practiced *Shokuiku* with him since he was born and that since learning of his ADHD diagnosis, she had limited his sugar intake a bit more and had increased his fish intake so he could get more of the healthy omega-3 fatty acids. After talking with her son's doctors and therapists and seeing how stable he had become after just six months of treatments, Motoko decided that the combination of all three—medication, therapy, and food—was what worked for him.

Motoko and her son's ADHD story is just one of many. There are a number of ways to treat ADHD in children and adults, just like there are a number of different levels of ADHD severity. Motoko doesn't claim to be an expert in the field of ADHD, but she is a mom of a child with ADHD and this diagnosis has impacted her life alongside her son's life. And while she believes in the power of nutrition and thinks food has helped her son, she also knows that her son absolutely needs medication and behavioral therapy too. As any parent would do for their child, she has found what works best for her son when it comes to treating his symptoms and improving his behavior.

Chapter 6

Bringing Your Family Together (and Saving Money)

Do you want to know how to simultaneously strengthen your family bond *and* teach your kids how to respect both you and their dinner? Of course you do, and food is the answer! Sharing meals with loved ones is about connecting to your family and your world.

Using all five senses at mealtimes will create vivid conversations and bring your family closer. **And the tradition of family togetherness during mealtimes, especially if established in early childhood, not only educates your child about food but fosters closeness and trust, and increases your child's social and emotional confidence all the way into their teen years.**[1]

For generations, Japanese families have been taking the time to show gratitude for their food, learning where their food comes from, and why certain foods taste the way they do. These cultural practices begin from an early age and happen as a family is gathered around the dining table together. Japanese families have found a stronger sense of togetherness and bonding from eating at least one meal per day together. And during this meal (or meals, for some families) there are rituals and traditions that occur that teach even the youngest family member to be thankful for their food and respectful of where the food comes from. Doesn't that sound amazing?

During family mealtimes, Japanese families come together and perform the following rituals that lead to closer connections:

- Prior to eating, the entire family says "*Itadamikasu*," which translates to "I will have / I will partake" and is also a request of "May I eat?" Saying *Itadamikasu* carries a meaning of gratitude to everything that happened to bring the food to the table as well as a sign of respect from the youngest family member to the oldest.

- When saying *Itadamikasu*, family members put their hands together as if praying. However, this is not a religious practice but a cultural one. Performing this physical act of putting their hands together helps each family member take a moment to appreciate the food and reflect inwardly.
- When the children have finished eating their meal, they say "*Gochisousamadeshita*," which means "*Thank you for the food, mom and dad.*" To *Gochisousamadeshita* the parents reply with either "*Yorosyu*" or "*Osomatsusama*," meaning "You're welcome" or "Well done."

While it's not necessary for your family to learn these Japanese words, we want to teach you how to take the time to truly honor where a meal comes from as well as the hands that make it. Even if they're your hands!

When children are taught to ask if they are allowed to eat before a meal and then thank their parents after they're done eating, they learn a high level of respect for both the food and their family. Respecting food and appreciating where it comes from is an important part of building a healthy relationship with food, an essential part of *Shokuiku*. Just think of how wonderful it would feel to be truly appreciated for putting food on the table every night!

HOW *SHOKUIKU* AND FAMILY MEALS SAVE MONEY

The average American child receives more than $6,500 worth of toys between the ages of 2 and 12.[2] Does this information shock you? Maybe, or maybe not. Whether you've spent this much, or more or less, on toys for your kids, you have not done anything wrong! Some parents may feel like they're buying new toys for their children almost continuously. Maybe this has happened to you when you see your child no longer playing with a once-beloved toy or becoming quickly bored with a new toy. It's only natural for you to want your kids to be happy, and new toys can bring a huge smile to your little one's face. But what if there were other more affordable ways for your child to be happy and entertained? And what if you could not only save money but also create fond memories and lifelong benefits for your entire family to look back on?

Shokuiku encourages families to view food as an adventure, where parents teach their children things like where each food on their plate comes from, what nutrients are in the meal, and why foods taste the way they do. These conversations can help kids learn more about the world and even decide for themselves if they truly enjoy certain foods or not. Japanese families practicing *Shokuiku* have also found that they can save money on toys and expensive classes because their family meals become an event and an educational adventure for their kids. Did you ever think that family meals could be the perfect time to share your knowledge with your kids and improve those bonds? You might even learn a few things yourself!

You may even be able to save money on expensive doctor visits and cold medicine for your entire family when you implement *Shokuiku.* When your family eats a wider variety of whole foods that are full of important nutrients and eat less of the processed foods that Americans are so used to, everyone under the roof can improve their health. Even making small changes in your child's diet, like regularly substituting a heavily processed school lunch with a fresh bento box, could mean fewer illnesses and trips to the doctor. And we know you might be thinking "Eating the *Shokuiku* way is going to cost me way more money!" But the trade-off will be the money you will save on your family's health.

TALKING WITH YOUR CHILDREN DURING FAMILY MEALS CAN IMPROVE RELATIONSHIPS

Did you know that talking with your children, including babies, during meals can help their brains develop and even improve their relationship with you? **Communication can make a meal much more enjoyable, and enjoying the mealtime experience may be just as important as the healthy foods on your plate!** Allowing your kids to be an active part of mealtime, including before, during, and after the meal, can foster family relationships and even improve your child's confidence (figure 6.1).[3]

Motoko's mother has helped her teach her son more about food by letting him help prepare meals and talking to him about the food they're making together. She has taught her grandson things like where rice comes from, how rice is grown, and all the people it takes to get rice from a farm to his plate. Motoko's mother and her son would also have conversations about cultures different from their own while eating new foods. Motoko also has plenty of dialog with her son while making food, like when they make "clumsy dumplings," or dumplings that don't look the traditional way, something she used to do when she was young. Her son will work hard on his dumpling for it to come out looking more like an abstract art piece than a dumpling. They'll laugh together and Motoko will encourage her son's efforts with words like "Wow, you made a soccer ball!"

Motoko's son would be fully engaged in these conversations and come away from them with loads of knowledge about food and respect for the foods he was about to eat. Plus, he had fun! Motoko's son also doesn't throw food away because he knows how valuable it is. He has learned from his mom and grandmother how much work goes into growing and making food. These conversations between Motoko's son and his elders make the entire family closer and enhance relationships. What a beautiful thing!

***

We hope these stories inspire you to start your own conversations with your family in the kitchen and around the dining table. Having conversations with family at every meal will help keep bonds strong and continuously growing. And having strong communication among family members can make for more engaging meals together for years. This can even be applied to those teenagers who tend to be of so few words. You may not always get a monolog from your 15-year-old son, but when focused conversations happen regularly around the table you can certainly get more than one-word answers, shoulder shrugs, or head nods when asking him about his day at school.

One great way to talk more with your kids while preparing or eating meals is to teach them about the different countries and cultures that made the meal's food popular. Motoko likes to use a globe to show her six-year-old son where countries and cultures can be found in the world. This teaches him just how big the world is and that there are many different cultures and types of foods to try. They even talk about geography during these conversations (and he is willing to do this outside of school!). His knowledge of new foods has led him to become quite the adventurous eater, even begging to try raw oysters on his sixth birthday. He loved them, by the way!

***

If you would rather try something else with your kids, you could consider learning about seasonal fruits and vegetables as a family. If you're not sure which fruits and vegetables are in season in your region throughout the year, you could search for and learn this information as a family. You could then use this knowledge when grocery shopping with your kids to find the

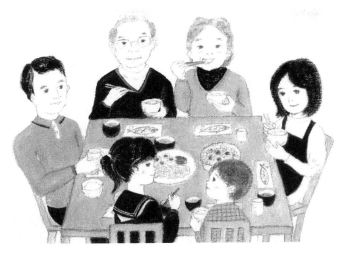

Figure 6.1 Family Dinner

freshest and most in-season produce for your dinners, making seeking out seasonal fruits and vegetables an opportunity for bonding. You could even go to a farmers' market or local farm with your kids to pick out fruits and vegetables that are in season. If you're not sure where to start, look at the fruits and vegetables your family already enjoys eating and find out when they are each in season. You may learn helpful things like avocados are in season in the winter, bananas are in season in the spring, carrots are in season in the summer, and apples are in season in the fall.

There is so much wonderful information to learn about produce besides the best seasons to eat them. You may learn when and how to harvest fruits and vegetables, why seasonal produce holds on to more nutrition than out-of-season produce, and even how to grow your own garden at home. You don't even need a backyard to grow your own food these days!

Americans are so used to being able to get any produce they want all year long (truly a luxury!) that they may not even realize that fruits and vegetables have seasons in which they taste better and are more nutritious. Fruits and vegetables that are in season when you buy them were grown during the best possible environment for them and are at their ripest and most delicious. Let's take spinach as an example. The best season for spinach to be harvested is the winter. Spinach tends to soak up the sun and take extra time going through photosynthesis steadily and slowly in the low winter temperatures. However, this slow process actually helps spinach store more high-quality nutrition. But when spinach is harvested in the summer under the harsh glare of the sun instead of its chosen season of winter, it absorbs more water faster than usual due to the heat. This causes the spinach to grow quicker than it would in the winter, but with less nutrition and taste. The winter spinach sounds so much better, doesn't it?

As a nutritionist, Marie is well-versed in the seasonal produce of Japan. And Motoko also has plenty of knowledge on the subject, since eating seasonal produce is common in Japan. Marie's 16-year-old nephew has been growing vegetables with his grandmother in her garden since he was very young. You would think a teenager would grow bored with this task, but he fully enjoys planting, watering, growing, and harvesting veggies to this day. He even enjoys helping his grandmother use his harvested veggies to prepare delicious and nutritious dishes. Marie has fond memories of watching her nephew have so much fun while taking beans out of the shell one-by-one when he was very little! Because her nephew and his grandmother were growing the vegetables themselves, they did not have to use fertilizers or pesticides. And, of course, they knew the right seasons to grow the different vegetables so they'd be the most delicious.

Marie has no doubt that growing your own produce is not as difficult as you may be thinking. Once you learn the right seasons to grow certain fruits and vegetables, you should have no trouble creating the right environment, temperature, or climate to help your crop thrive!

There are so many benefits to growing your own fruits and vegetables, like higher nutritional value and having a sense of peace from knowing exactly where your food comes from. And your kids will love it! They will enjoy picking out seeds, taking care of the plants, and eventually harvesting and eating their very own fruits and vegetables, all with you by their side.

***

As you can imagine, there is much more to discuss regarding healthy, whole foods than ultra-processed foods. A conversation about how fresh crops are grown, picked, and manufactured before arriving in your grocery store aisles or how different cultures prepare foods special to them would be enlightening, interesting, and enjoyable. But you probably would *not* enjoy a conversation about the steps it takes to produce foods made in factories with the help of lots of sugar, salt, and synthetic ingredients. Here's an example of what we mean: Fresh produce is simply plucked from the ground and cleaned before it is ready to eat, while hot dogs are made by turning leftover pieces of pork, beef, and chicken (they use *all* the body parts . . . like feet!) into a mystery slime that is eventually put into casings made of collagen then fully cooked long before actually making their way into your hands.

When you gather around and discuss a healthy meal you are about to eat, your entire family will nourish both their bodies and their minds. A well-nourished child will be more active (in a good way!) and may even elicit more meaningful interactions from their parents.[4] These interactions could come full circle back to the dinner table and continue on over years of adventurous meals that bring families closer together.

You can foster great family relationships by asking your children to help you prepare the food and include them in the conversations that occur around the dining table. It doesn't matter how old your child is—even one-way conversations with your baby can help build healthy relationships with food and each other, even if they are babbling their comments back to you! There are so many wonderful things to talk about during meals, like how the food was made, the culture from where the food comes from, why we eat it, and even why foods look and taste different. **By simply bringing your children into the mealtime conversation you can develop a strong tie and provide stability and security, no matter their age.** Trust starts at birth, and with a solid foundation of communication, you will see your child open up to you throughout their lives (even those moody teen years)!

WHY IT'S IMPORTANT TO ELIMINATE DISTRACTIONS DURING MEALS

Has your family fallen into the common-these-days habit of being distracted by phones, social media, toys, or TV during meals? Whether your family uses devices during meals or not, the fact of the matter is that phones can't bring you the true happiness and feelings of connection that conversation and bonding during a meal can. This probably won't come as a surprise, but fairly recent research has shown that phone use during a meal leads to more distraction and less enjoyment of the meal and people around them.[5] In a time where more and more kids (and their parents) are growing up with an electronic device by their side, it's imperative for families to make an extra effort to stay close.

If you're ready to have more meaningful meals with your family, the final step may be to eliminate devices and distractions during those meals. Just remember "The D's": No **D**evices or **D**istractions during **D**inner. You will find that once you make a rule about devices and distraction at the dinner table that both you and your children are happier and better nourished. Eliminating mealtime distractions could improve your family's health and nutrition. And when there are no devices allowed at dinner, you will have no choice but to talk to your family!

Food is meant to be more than just nutrition. There are social, emotional, and even spiritual components of food, and participating in family meals can expand and promote these. Think about special meals and holidays gathered around a fancy dining room table. Why are these so special and memorable? These meals are especially memorable because of not only the delicious food that is usually present but also the conversations, laughs, and smiles shared with loved ones (we all have at least one hilarious, emotional, or embarrassing story from a big family dinner).

But there is no rule that says these types of special, distraction-free meals can't happen any time of the year and not just on holidays. As humans, we crave and require social interaction, and this starts from the time we are babies. When children actively and socially participate in family meals, they tend to begin to mimic eating choices, patterns, and behaviors modeled by family members.[6] **This means you, the parent, must eat and behave as you want your child to while at the dinner table.** As much as you might want to eat their dino nuggets, if your child sees you eating fast food while watching TV when they instead have a plate of fresh fruits and vegetables in front of them and no show, they will want to be like you and may only eat once you hand over some chips!

Family mealtimes nourish more than just your bodies. A family feeding environment includes physical, social, and emotional interactions between family members that nourish not only your family's bodies but also their minds, spirits, and hearts.[7] You may be wondering how food can be a spiritual experience. Well, when you have conversations about where your food comes from, you become more appreciative of it and can start to build a spiritual connection with food. This could include taking the time to talk with your family about who planted the seeds of the spinach in your salad or where the salmon on top of your salad was caught. Then, you could talk about what the food tastes like or how it will nourish your body (for example, protein can help build muscle and healthy fats can help your brain). Humans have an innate connection to nature, and spirituality, and no matter what your religion is, it can be a big part of gratitude and connectedness to life.

You can also build spiritual connections around meals that have special meaning to your family, like a recipe passed down from a grandmother or a cooking technique taught by your great-uncle. Think about how wonderful it would feel to prepare a meal your grandmother used to make for you for your family, then watch them enjoy that meal while sharing stories and memories. Simply being present with both your food and your family during meals can foster a spiritual relationship that enhances the mealtime experience.

OSECHI, A BEAUTIFUL JAPANESE NEW YEAR'S MEAL

A great example of how meals can become more than meals occurs on New Year's Day in Japan. On the first of January, families come together and enjoy a very special meal at home. This meal is called *Osechi* and it has a rich history.

Osechi dates all the way back to the AD 700s when festivals were held five times per year at the imperial court, one for each time the seasons changed and one for New Year's Day. Through the centuries, these festivals evolved and eventually became a celebration for all Japanese people and not just the nobles. And over time, the celebration became focused solely on New Year's Day and this is how *Osechi* became the special meal throughout Japanese homes that it is to this day.

The *Osechi* meal itself is pretty extravagant and can take hours to days to prepare. You might compare it to America's Thanksgiving, with family members all gathering for one day of cooking, eating, and enjoying each other's company as they look forward to the new year. In the past, the foods prepared for *Osechi* were made with lots of salt and other preservatives so that they could be eaten as leftovers for a few days and give moms and homemakers a much-deserved break. Fortunately, refrigerators were invented and now the many foods prepared for *Osechi* can be fresh, whole foods often enjoyed in Japan. As many as 20 to 30 different dishes may be made for *Osechi* for just one family. Now you can see why the meal takes so long to prepare!

Osechi is not something you will find on a Japanese restaurant menu in America, as it is a meal that is meant to be enjoyed by a family and in the family home. Even the way the foods are arranged and presented is meaningful. Foods are placed in boxes called *Jubako* that are similar to bento boxes but different because they are tiered (figure 6.2). The tiers allow foods to be packed in layers, and multiple *Jubakos* can be stacked on each other to symbolize the piling up of good luck and fortune in the new year. The foods inside each box have special meanings too (more on this soon). Some Japanese families even take the time to make elaborate designs and

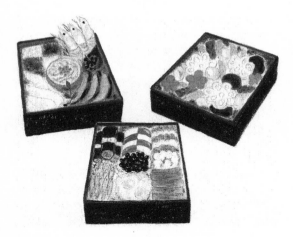

Figure 6.2   Osechi

decorations out of the food they will enjoy on New Year's Day. These
boxes are truly beautiful!

Like many of the Japanese family meals enjoyed together, *Osechi* is
a way for families to come together without distractions from their busy
lives. In this way, they can enjoy each other's company and share the
beginning of the new year together. Marie has fond memories of bonding
with her nephew while preparing foods for *Osechi*. It typically takes her
about 15 hours to prepare *Osechi,* an exhausting but rewarding feat! Her
nephew often watches her prepare the meal and will talk with her about the
different foods and customs surrounding *Osechi*. This extra involvement on
his part has made Marie's nephew more excited to eat the foods he helped
bring to the table on New Year's Day. He even hopes to share what he has
learned from Marie with his kids in the future. How sweet!

Foods made for *Osechi* may vary a bit from region to region in Japan,
but the meanings behind many of the foods are the same all over the country. Popular and meaningful *Osechi* foods include:

Ebi: *Ebi* (shrimp) is often used in *Osechi* to wish for a long life, even after
your back has bent over like a shrimp's.
Kikkakabu: The chrysanthemum, or *kiku,* one of the national flowers
of Japan, represents longevity. For *Osechi,* some turnips are cut up
to resemble the shape of a *kiku* flower. They are seasoned with sweet
vinegar.

Kuromame: *Mame* means "bean," but it can also be used to describe someone who works diligently, as *mame* originally meant "good health and strength" in Japanese. Japanese people eat *Kuromame (black soybeans)* on New Year's Day, wishing for longevity and saying "May we be healthy and spend days diligently all year-round."

Chorogi: *Chorogi* (Chinese artichoke) is marinated in red Japanese plum vinegar, and it is used in *Osechi* as a lucky charm garnished with *Kuromame*. Since it is written with the Japanese characters for Long, Old, and Happiness (長老喜), it describes longevity. Eaten with *Kuromame,* which represents good health, the dish as a whole describes people's wishes to stay healthy and to live long.

Tatsukuri: Also known as *Gomame, Tatsukuri* is a dish of small crispy sardines seasoned with sugar, soy sauce, and sweet sake. The name *Tatsukuri* literally means "rice farming" and it comes from the custom of using baby sardines in fields as fertilizer, wishing for a good harvest.

Kurikinton: A favorite dish for kids on New Year's Day, *Kurikinton* translates to "chestnut gold mash" and is made of mashed Japanese sweet potatoes and chestnuts that have been candied in syrup. Japanese sweet potatoes are starchier and sweeter than traditional sweet potatoes. This sweet dish represents economic fortune and wealth in the upcoming year.

Kazunoko: *Kazunoko* is made from herring roe (or small fish eggs) that have been marinated in *Dashi*, or soy sauce and soup stock. This dish is described as a delicacy with a salty and savory flavor and a lovely golden yellow color. *Kazunoko* symbolizes a prosperous family with many children.

Kobumaki: This *Osechi* dish contains the Japanese word for happiness, *kobu*, and as such it wishes happiness and luck in the new year. *Kobumaki* is sea kelp (or *Konbu*) rolled then cooked in a sweet, savory sauce. Sometimes these rolls are tied shut with *Kanpyo*, or strips of dried gourd.

While American families may not make 20 to 30 dishes for New Year's Day (or any day, for that matter), they may be able to take something from *Osechi*. You could let *Osechi* inspire you to make a special, celebratory meal for the new year, or any joyous occasion. Perhaps there is a holiday you wish your family celebrated with a meal or knew more about. **Next time that holiday comes around, you could learn more about it and then share what you learned with your family as you prepare a special**

meal together. But these learning and teaching moments don't have to only take place around holidays. As we have been saying, there are many ways to connect with your family throughout the mealtime experience. Remember, you don't need a garden to help your child be more excited to eat vegetables (but it certainly might help!). Simply teaching them where the veggies they are about to eat comes from might spark their interest enough for them to eat them, or at least give them a try!

Chapter 7

Fighting Disease and Childhood Obesity

America has one of the highest obesity rates in the world (66% of its population is obese or overweight according to BMI).[1] And while BMI, or Body Mass Index, isn't always the best tool to use when analyzing body compositions, the truth remains that many American families don't have nutritious diets.[2] But not all hope is lost.

If you ever visit Japan, you will probably notice that most people walking on the sidewalk are not fat (you'll definitely notice this as an American!). We know from research that Japanese children are fed one of the best diets in the world, as their parents set them up for long, healthy lives from an early age. Using the many old Japanese wisdoms of *Shokuiku*, you can set your children up to be healthier adults. One method in particular called *Hara Hachi Bun Me*, or eating until 80% full, may be the secret to helping your children keep their disease risk low, and it doesn't cost a thing (more on this later)! The habits created now while they're children will last a lifetime (as do their fat cells if Americans continue the pattern of unhealthy eating).[3]

It's easy in the day-to-day business of our lives to forget how powerful food is, but it has the ability to make or break your overall health. You don't have to be a nutritionist to learn the basics of nutrition and how to properly feed yourself and your family in a way that improves your health, decreases your risk for many health issues, and increases longevity. Hippocrates said it best: "Let food be thy medicine and thy medicine be food."

OBESITY STATISTICS AND WHY
NUTRITION IS SO IMPORTANT

Obesity isn't a disease itself, but as you probably know, being overweight can come with a high risk of developing many potentially fatal diseases like heart disease and diabetes, no matter your age. **The harsh reality is that parents are fully responsible for the health of their children, so how you approach food and feeding your child from day one matters.** Alarmingly, the number of children in the United States who are overweight has doubled since the 1960s. Basically, kids today are bigger than their parents' and grandparents' generations. The single biggest cause of a child being overweight is how, what, and when parents feed their kids.[4]

As unfair as it may seem, if your child becomes overweight in the early years of their life, this can negatively affect their physical and mental health as adults. Did you know that the number of fat cells you have for the rest of your life is set when you are still a child?[5] That's right, your food and activity behaviors as a child have the potential to haunt you as an adult. However, even though you can't change the number of fat cells you have in your body over time, you can change their density, as they shrink with weight loss and increase with weight gain. When you lose weight, you don't lose fat cells, you simply shrink them so they can't hold as much fat. But this is reversible, meaning these fat cells can easily regrow and regain the capacity to hold on to more fat.

It's truly easy to unintentionally overfeed your child or feed him too many foods high in added sugar and extra calories. It's also easy to be much too fearful of food and feeding your child, leading to restricting food from your child, which can cause disordered eating habits and even eating disorders for years to come. Basically, parenting is hard! But we're here to talk about the all-too-common issue in America of childhood obesity and what you as a parent can do to help your child not become a statistic.

Overeating is a big issue with American children, with the rates of overweight and obesity increasing 10 to 15% in children between the ages of 2 and 19.[6] Although diseases do not automatically come along with being categorized as overweight or even obese, this population of children in America is at a higher risk for medical issues like type 2 diabetes, hypertension, and obstructive sleep apnea, on top of other issues like poor self-esteem, disturbed body image, depression, and eating disorders.[7] Not to mention the unfair and sad but true fact that overweight and obese children often face social stigmatization from their classmates due to their body size.

***

In Japan, the prevalence of childhood obesity is low, especially compared to countries like the United States. Much of this is attributed to the success of the school lunch program (*Kyushoku*) you learned about in chapter 5. There have even been studies on how the lower rate of childhood obesity in Japan is at least partly due to *Kyushoku* and the well-balanced, nourishing lunches that are a part of that program.[8] However, mostly due to the COVID pandemic, lockdowns, and more time being spent away from school, Japanese children seem to be gradually gaining weight.

Marie has also grown concerned for the number of children in her country who are being left to eat alone by busy parents. These kids tend to eat more processed foods, sugar, and carbohydrates that tend to be culprits of obesity and other issues like diabetes if regularly eaten in excess. Marie only wishes these parents understood that they have the power to help their children learn how to properly nourish their bodies when left to eat alone. She feels many parents in both Japan and America simply don't know how to feed their children in a healthier way. It's a lack of nutrition education.

While overweight children have always existed, the prevalence of children categorized as overweight or obese has certainly increased over recent years. **As of 2020, there were 39 million children under the age of 5 and more than 340 million children aged 5 to 19 who were categorized as overweight or obese all around the world.**[9] And while there can be many factors that go into a child being overweight or obese, environmental influences are at least partially to blame.[10]

Young children just can't make the best choices when it comes to their nutrition, at least not without proper nutrition education and understanding of why what they eat matters. And American schools and governments fail parents significantly here.

A child's metabolism may be higher than their parents, but that doesn't mean they should be able to eat freely or overindulge on chicken nuggets and candy. But restricting your child's food, having your child go on an official "diet," or having strict food rules in your house can also be detrimental, as excessive control in feeding your child has been linked to poorer eating regulation, and thus increased body weight.[11] So what is the middle ground? Enter *Shokuiku*.

We tell you all these somewhat scary facts and statistics not only to alert your attention, but also because there is still plenty of time for you and your family to make positive changes that can help you all have longer and healthier lives. **And the first step is to establish new behaviors around food that will lead to sustainable lifestyle changes.**

HOW THE WESTERN DIET HAS
CHANGED HEALTH IN JAPAN

Obesity rates for both children and adults in Japan are drastically lower than those of Americans, but they are slowly creeping up. Like many other Japanese people, Marie and Motoko think things started to change when fast food and the Western diet were introduced to the country. And, unfortunately, America was the country to introduce these. We know convenience foods are much higher in calories, saturated fat, and added sugar than fresh, whole foods. But they are just that, convenient. Instead, taking just a bit of extra time to prepare meals and snacks made from nutrient-dense ingredients can have a major impact on your health.

As someone who has split her time living between Japan and the United States, Motoko has seen the differences in food choices and obesity first-hand. One of the places she always sees the most glaringly obvious difference between the two countries is at the beloved Disneyland. As you know, people from all over the United States and even all over the world come to visit the magical Disneyland. But Motoko can't help but notice the number of children and adults she sees sitting and eating large treats rather than walking around and truly enjoying the park (figure 7.1). She'll see kids old enough to be walking instead being pushed in a wagon while eating an ice cream cone bigger than their head! Or she'll see entire families needing frequent breaks from walking through the park. And these breaks seem to always entail a new sweet treat. These sights make Motoko feel sad that these families are unable to see and enjoy Disneyland as they should. If only they had been properly fueling and moving their bodies regularly, they may have been able to experience all of Disneyland.

The story of the people of Okinawa is one more example of how Western culture has influenced some of the people of Japan's eating habits. You already know that Japanese people tend to live longer than many people in the rest of the world. But in Japan, the people living on the island of Okinawa live even longer. The longer life span of the people of Okinawa is attributed to their diet, which is very high in vegetables and low in fat and calories. The diet also focuses on soy products for protein and some other foods like rice and fish, but is mostly made up of low-glycemic carbohydrates. However, even Okinawa is not immune to the Western diet. There is now a military base on Okinawa where Americans live. Once the Americans arrived, there was new interest in foods like hamburgers and fries on the island. Obviously, hamburgers don't quite fit in with the traditional healthy Okinawa diet!

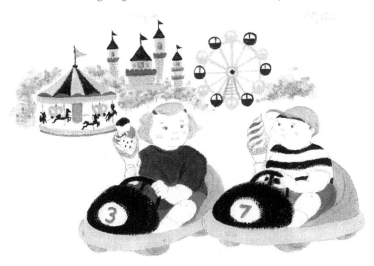

Figure 7.1 A boy eating icecream in a cart at a theme park

FOOD AS MEDICINE

As we said at the top of this chapter, food can be used as medicine. Many foods are full of powerful nutrients that can fight off diseases, help you maintain your weight, and fuel your body for sports, recreation, or just getting through the day. The steps to a healthier and longer life are simpler than you may think, and you don't need to go on the latest fad diet to achieve health—in fact, you might do more harm than good with some of those diets!

There is no big secret to nutrition. The facts are simple: You need to eat plenty of foods that are high in nutrition to get all the nutrients your body needs for optimal health while limiting the foods that don't do much for your health, like ultra-processed meals and snacks, sweets, and sugary beverages. Fortunately, you do not have to cut the fun foods completely out of your or your child's diet to be healthy. We completely understand there are birthday parties and dinners at friends' houses and meals on the road. Plus, when you restrict something completely it will only make you or your child want it more!

This is where *Shokuiku* comes in. Whether you've been trying to think of ways to improve your family's nutrition for a while and have come up short, or you're just now realizing that some changes need to be made, or

you're still in the contemplation phase, you can apply the principles of
Shokuiku to turn your family's health around and set your children up for
the future.

Don't worry, you don't have to be like Buddhist monks to follow
Shokuiku. Although, some of their eating habits are extremely healthy and
we can take some notes from them! For example, *Shojin-ryori* is a cultural
style of healthy eating made popular by Japanese Buddhist monks. It entails
eating meals made without meat, fish, or any animal products at all. It's
essentially veganism, but the meaning behind it is deeper. Buddhist tradition did not allow the killing of animals for human consumption, as this
was thought to interfere with daily meditations.[12] To make up for the lack of
animal foods, *Shojin-ryori* typically includes tofu or other soy products as
well as plenty of seasonal vegetables. However, these days a *Shojin-ryori*
meal may include dairy products, as Buddhist monks feel that getting milk
from a cow is not harmful.[13] Spices are used sparingly, as they are thought
to mask the true flavor of the fresh foods. In a nutshell, *Shojin-ryori* is an
eating style that is both cultural and spiritual and can be practiced by anyone who wants to, not just Buddhist monks.

HOW *SHOKUIKU* CAN HELP LOWER DISEASE RISKS AND IMPROVE HEALTH FOR THE ENTIRE FAMILY

The children of Japan are expected to live longer than those in any other
country, with an average life span of 83 years.[14] The Japanese lifestyle,
including eating the *Shokuiku* way and staying physically active, is a testament to the longevity of its citizens. And, as you've been learning in the
previous chapters, working toward a longer life begins as soon as Japanese
children enter the world. As they grow up, the children of Japan are taught
to eat the food that is put before them by their parents or elders, which
leads to children being more likely to accept rather than reject or even have
a tantrum over the food they are given.[15] What this translates to is Japanese
children regularly consuming highly nutritious meals that the meal preparer
has put time and thought into to make it balanced.

**This regular eating of nutrient-dense foods from a young age helps
the Japanese population ward off diseases like cancer, type 2 diabetes,
heart disease, and neurodegenerative diseases.** And eating the *Shokuiku*
way can even help improve sleep, another important factor in reducing
disease risk.[16] The improvements in sleep alone should be enough for any
seemingly always tired parent to try *Shokuiku*!

One of the healthiest diets in the world is the Japanese diet, which contains about five times the amount of cancer-fighting cruciferous vegetables (like bok choy, cabbage, broccoli, and cauliflower) as the typical American diet.[17] Cruciferous veggies are beneficial in many ways, including slowing down certain enzymes that can feed carcinogens or helping other enzymes that can destroy carcinogens.[18] In this way, eating as the Japanese do will reduce your family's risk of cancer.

But the people of Japan are doing much more than eating more cruciferous vegetables to keep some of their disease rates lower than those in America. They're also limiting their intake of saturated fat, salt, and added sugar while focusing on eating plenty of fish containing omega-3 fatty acids, soy (plant-based proteins), antioxidant-rich foods and drinks, and other whole foods like fruits, vegetables, and whole grains.[19]

With only 4.8% of Japanese men and 3.7% of Japanese women being categorized as obese,[20] these low statistics are thought to contribute to the lower rates of diseases like cancer and some types of heart disease in Japan as well.[21] And since we know that carrying extra weight can increase the risk of many diseases, it's important to find a healthy weight for your body so you too can decrease your disease risk. But you still don't need any expensive diet or cleanse to help you and your family achieve healthy body weights.

Another condition that may be able to be fixed with better nutrition is insomnia. Wait, what? Better sleep? Moms and dads, we see your ears perk up, and yes! ***Shokuiku* principles can help you and your child sleep more soundly as well.** Better sleep will help everyone in the house feel better and more energized during the day. But many health conditions can also derive from not getting quality sleep. You may be able to avoid conditions like diabetes, hypertension, obesity, and mood disorders with healthy Z's.[22] But besides helping parents, *Shokuiku* can also help lower your child's risk of developing sleep disorders like insomnia. Scientists discovered that kids who eat fish one or more times a week sleep better and score higher on IQ tests. Omega-3s, the fatty acids found in foods like fatty fish and walnuts, are connected with better sleep, which also translated into higher intelligence by about five points according to one Chinese study of over 500 kids.[23] And since eating the *Shokuiku* way will involve a higher intake of fish containing omega-3 fatty acids, your kids and your family are sure to reap the benefits of better sleep!

Better nutrition can also protect and improve brain health. One large analysis of several studies found that those who ate more fruits and vegetables had significantly lower risks of cognitive decline (things like memory loss, trouble learning new things, and concentration) and dementia.[24] People following *Shokuiku* consume a variety of fruits and vegetables that contain powerful antioxidants and other nutrients thought to protect the brain and all its important functions. Other foods thought to contain brain-protective nutrients like antioxidants and healthy fats include dark leafy greens, fatty fish, and tea—foods that are commonly eaten regularly in Japan.

Eating the *Shokuiku* way can help keep disease risk low. *Shokuiku* focuses on foods that are rich in vitamins, minerals, omega-3 fatty acids, fiber, antioxidants, and other nutrients, and this can help you and your child maintain a healthy body weight. These foods (and others!) will also help your family fight off potentially harmful substances that make their way into your bodies. It's important to remember, though, that the nutrients and foods we've been talking about here need to be eaten regularly and as part of an overall healthy, nutritious diet to reap the benefits. Basically, there are no magic foods that can solve all the health problems of your family if eaten just once. Sorry! But you can make positive and sustainable lifestyle changes that will have an impact. *Shokuiku* is one of these sustainable options since it's not a tough-to-follow fad diet. It's not a diet at all! At least not in the way you may be thinking. Instead, *Shokuiku* is a way of life that can be followed forever and help you keep your risk of many diseases low and have longevity.

HARA HACHI BUN ME

In chapter 5, you read about how school lunches in Japan (*Kyushoku*) are superior to American school lunches and are helping the country keep its rates of childhood obesity and other diseases low. The success of *Kyushoku* is thought to stem from many aspects of the very nutritious school lunches, like how the meals are made with fresh foods on-site (in America, many of the lunch items arrive at the schools frozen, packaged, or in other preserved forms) or how, unlike in America, there are no vending machines in Japanese schools that students can run to for an afternoon snack after an unsatisfying lunch, leaving Japanese students more likely to finish their entire satisfying lunch provided by their school.[25]

But there are other aspects of Japanese culture and *Shokuiku* that better set their children up for a long, healthy life than many other countries, including the United States. *Hara Hachi Bun Me* is another Japanese term often repeated in *Shokuiku* teachings. This phrase roughly translates to "Eat until you are 80% full" and comes from the tradition of Confucianism that

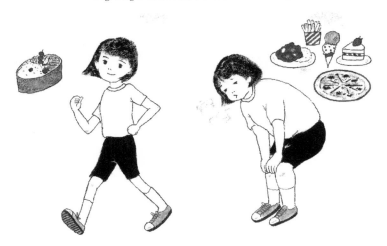

Figure 7.2   Eating full vs eating 80%

encourages eating moderate-sized portions (figure 7.2).[26] *Hara Hachi Bun Me* helps people eat meals for the purpose of satisfaction and nourishment and not for walking away from the dining table feeling incredibly full and uncomfortable. We all know that feeling!

Hara Hachi Bun Me is widely used throughout Japan and it's a phrase parents often tell their kids during meals. When your family eats in this way, you can all start to appreciate the taste of your food more while also reducing your risk for diseases that can pop up when carrying around extra weight. Your family can start working on figuring out what 80% full feels like by eating meals more slowly and allowing your brain to catch up with your stomach and send signals of satiety, or satisfaction from food. When practicing this method, it's best to stop eating when you and your kids just start feeling full. This will help prevent everyone from overeating. It's also helpful to slow down and chew bites of food several times. Better-chewed food is easier to digest, which means more nutrients can be absorbed and used by the body.

You and your kids could even try eating with chopsticks, which require more effort and intention to use and automatically slow down a meal (using them has even been linked to lower obesity rates).[27] Can you imagine the laughs around the table when your kids try to use chopsticks for the first time? And slowing down will be easy when you and your family are practicing *Shokuiku*, since you will be having meaningful conversations about the food you are eating anyway!

It can be challenging to stop eating sometimes, especially when the food is tasting great and you are having fun eating it. When you and your kids start incorporating *Hara Hachi Bun Me*, you can remind them of something many elderly people in Japan like to say near the end of meals. When they start feeling full from their meal, Japanese elders will say something like "That looks very good to eat but I think I'll stop here." They'll say this because they know it's more important to listen to their body's cues about being satisfied from the meal, even though eating the rest of the food in front of them sounds enjoyable.

The basic point is this: Just because there is food that tastes good in front of you doesn't mean you have to eat it! Part of living a healthier and longer life is learning to listen to your body and honor your hunger and satiety cues. And you and your family can do this by slowing down during meals, allowing your brain time to catch up with your stomach, and learning how to eat until 80% full. We promise you'll still walk away from a meal feeling satisfied when you eat in this way!

GIVE ONLY WHAT THEY'LL EAT!

When Motoko's son fills up his self-serve yogurt, she reminds him of another Japanese food philosophy, "Take only what you can eat." Historically, there was no "buffet culture" in Japan, whereas Americans seem to get a thrill over how high the food stacks on their plates that will probably never make it to their stomach (if it does, it will cause uncomfortable fullness anyway). In Japan, it is shameful to take excessive food that ends up being wasted. This is called *Mottainai*, meaning "What a waste!" and is extremely frowned on. The solution is not to gorge on the food you get, but to only get what your body truly needs. This teaches self-regulation from an early age.

But parents can also have their own saying, "Give only what they'll eat." Rather than giving your child the entire bag of popcorn, try giving them a portion of it in their own special, small bowl. Having an entire bag of snacks in your grasp can easily lead to mindless eating, especially if you're doing something else at the same time. And this can happen for kids as well as adults. How many times has your child sat in front of the TV with a bag of chips or box of cookies and eaten so much they have no room for their nutritious dinner? When snacks are portioned by you, the knowledgeable parent, you can cut down on a lot of waste. And we mean both the waste of the yummy, healthy foods you made for dinner your kid can't eat because they're stuffed and the waste of money on having to buy new bags of popcorn all the time!

Speaking of kids having snacks in front of the TV, remember the section on eliminating distractions in the last chapter? Both kids and adults can easily fall victim to digital distractions. It's easy to get sucked into a good show or social media post! But eliminating distractions is important, not only for meals but also for snacks. It will be much easier to practice principles of *Shokuiku* (like *Hara Hachi Bun Me* and "Take only what you'll eat") when you and your kids eat undistracted. Distractions tend to lead to more overeating and mindless eating due to paying attention to the screen instead of the plate.

Using small bowls and plates is customary in Japan and is just another way that helps families there keep both weight and disease risk low. And what they put in those small dishes obviously contributes to their glowing health statistics. *Ichiju Sansai* translates to "one soup, three dishes" and is how Japanese meals are structured. There is always one soup or liquid dish that is consumed at the start of the meal. Drinking a dish first helps prevent overeating, as the liquid will immediately fill your stomach and give you a bit of satisfaction.

After the soup portion of the meal, the next phase of *Ichiju Sansai* is three small dishes plus a small side of rice (figure 7.3). As you learned in chapter 4, all food is put on the table at the same time and in separate dishes to promote the Triangle method of eating in a round-robin fashion. You may recall that the Triangle method also helps people slow down while eating because it allows extra time to think about what you are about to eat. The entrees and sides are all put on small plates or in small bowls to keep portions moderate. And the foods eaten typically include several vegetable options, lean protein like fish or tofu, and steamed rice. Some Japanese families will eat the vegetables first to improve digestion and make sure they get those important nutrients in before moving on to the other foods before them. Eating fiber-rich veggies first also helps prevent big blood sugar spikes and instead allows blood sugar to rise much slower.

And don't forget to aim for a variety of foods at each meal, especially vegetables. Veggies are packed with so many wonderful nutrients that can help fight off diseases. Motoko can't help but notice that when she asks for a salad or extra veggies at a restaurant, what's brought out almost every time is broccoli, and only broccoli! Of course, broccoli is a nutrient-packed veggie option, but there are plenty of other great options that should also be offered. The more the merrier when it comes to vegetable variety.

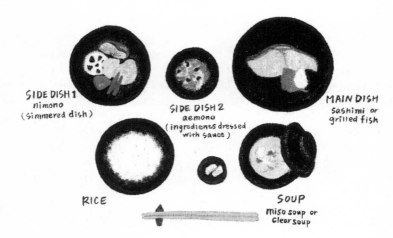

Figure 7.3   Ichiju Sansai

Following Japanese eating methods of only putting out what you actually need to eat in small dishes, eating soup and veggies first, eating with chopsticks, eating a wider variety of foods, and using the Triangle method are all tactics that can help you and your family take steps toward reducing disease risks. Your family can also follow healthy Japanese eating traditions like putting utensils down between bites or while talking to encourage slow eating. And, as you now know, eating slowly and chewing thoroughly helps prevent overeating.

FEEDING YOUR CHILDREN TO HELP
REDUCE THEIR DISEASE RISK

So, how can you apply all this information to feeding your children and reducing their risk of various diseases? Well, you can start with posture. You weren't expecting that, were you? American parents may ask their kids to remove their elbows from the table or stop playing with their food for the sake of good behavior during meals (important and reasonable asks!), but posture while eating is not always a topic of conversation. However, how you and your kids sit while eating actually affects how the food is digested,[28] and good digestion means better utilization of nutrients that can then go on to help the body fight off illness and disease.

You don't need a deep knowledge of human anatomy to understand that eating, say, lying down would be problematic. Well, eating with poor posture with your back bent and stomach crunched also does not give your digestive system the space it needs to work properly. Instead, work with your kids on sitting close to the table with their backs straight, knees bent at a 90-degree angle, and, preferably, with their feet on a flat surface, like the floor, stool, or foot tray on a highchair.

Besides posture, there are plenty of fairly simple changes you can make to your child's diet to improve their health. Like you learned in chapter 3, *Shokuiku* starts from a young age, and how you feed your baby or toddler matters for their health, development, and growth. Besides not feeding their babies processed foods when starting solids, Japanese parents also avoid giving their tots sauces and dips with foods, and this helps the children grow to enjoy the taste of simple foods, which can stay with them. Of course, you can gradually introduce sauces and bolder flavors to your kids as they grow up, but adding these on the side of dishes will allow your child to explore flavors on their own and use less of them, which is a good thing since many dips tend to be high in things like calories and added sugar that kids don't need.

As we have been saying all along, giving your kids a variety of healthy foods is best. Trying new foods regularly can help eliminate picky eaters. You can even give your babies that are just starting solid foods common allergens now—in fact, it's recommended! This means you can let your baby try foods like peanuts or peanut butter, shellfish, wheat, and eggs around six months of age (but make sure your pediatrician gives you the green light first), and this should help reduce their risk of developing an allergy to these foods.[29]

PROCESSED FOODS AND ADDED SUGAR

It's important to remember the keyword *healthy* when giving your child new foods to try. It's practically a given that kids will like salty snacks and sugary treats immediately, but it's the nutritious foods like fruits, vegetables, whole grains, and fish that you want to make sure they develop a hankering for, or at least enjoy! It may sound tricky, but if you can keep your child away from foods containing added sugar for the first year, this can help develop their palate immensely. We all know that sugar tastes good, but if you give your six-month-old ice cream as one of his first foods, it's going to be tough for him to accept those mushed carrots that are coming up next. And which would you rather him have? The carrots, of course!

Feeding your kids the *Shokuiku* way means avoiding added sugar and processed foods for a while as they grow accustomed to the more nutritious stuff. How many parents hear this when their kids sit down to dinner: "Ew, green things! How many do I have to eat?" And thus ensues a dinnertime battle to wear on every parent's nerve. Motoko's son gladly eats his vegetables first, without a fight.

But, obviously, you can't and don't need to have your kids avoid sugar forever. That's just plain cruel! Restriction only causes problems anyway. So, what are you as a parent supposed to do with the whole added sugar and ultra-processed foods dilemma? Instead of avoiding these foods, a better word to use is *limit*. This involves making sure kids eat plenty of nutrient-dense foods first and most often but allowing treats and fun foods here and there. It's important to limit calorie-dense foods like sweets and salty snacks so that your child has plenty of room in her belly for all the nutrients she needs to grow and develop. In case you are wondering, it is recommended that kids consume no more than 2,300 mg of sodium (or salt) and 25 grams or less of added sugar in a day.[30]

Here are a few more helpful tips when it comes to processed snacks and added sugar for kids:

- Sugar added to food can go by many names on a food label. Look out for words like dextrose, brown sugar, cane sugar, corn sweetener, corn syrup, evaporated cane juice, fructose sweetener, honey, maple syrup, molasses, isomalt, maltodextrin, mannitol, rice syrup solids, sorbitol, concentrated fruit juice, and, of course, high-fructose corn syrup, among others.[31]
- You can find out how much added sugar is in a food by looking at the nutrition facts label. This will be listed on the line titled "Includes X Grams of Added Sugars," with the number filled in for X being the number of grams of added sugar inside one serving of the food.
- Ultra-processed foods will often list many types of added sugar as well as other unrecognizable ingredients on the nutrition label. What makes a food ultra-processed is the fact that it is made with ingredients like synthetic flavors, sweeteners, and additives that will help the food last longer. Basically, ultra-processed foods are not fresh.
- These highly processed foods also contain high levels of sodium and fat that are known to lead to health issues and diseases like type 2 diabetes and heart disease if regularly eaten in excess.

- Examples of ultra-processed foods include frozen meals, hot dogs, packaged snacks (flavored potato chips, cookies, many types of crackers), prepared cakes, soft drinks, candy, instant noodles and other instant meals, sugary cereals, and energy drinks.

Although eating processed foods and added sugar from time and time is okay and won't immediately damage your child's health, eating too much of these foods can set them up for the potential to develop the diseases and disorders we've been talking about, like type 2 diabetes, sleep disorders, and heart disease. Eating lots of sugar and not enough nutritious foods can also throw your gut and digestion out of whack. You've probably seen commercials or heard advertisements for probiotics that are meant to restore the good bacteria in your gut. But how can bacteria be good? Aren't we trying to avoid it? Well, in general, yes, but you and your kids actually need a balance of good and bad bacteria in your digestive tract for proper digestion and absorption of nutrients. However, it's pretty easy for these bacteria in your gut to become off-balance, with there being more of the bad guys than the good guys in there. This can happen with a diet high in things like added sugar, sodium, and saturated fat. Fortunately, your entire family can restore their gut health with plenty of healthy foods and some extra probiotics from fermented foods like sugar-free Greek yogurt, tempeh, and kombucha (If you want to try Japanese fermented foods, you can try using soy sauce and miso which are the common tasty condiments of Japan).

When you keep your gut health in check, you keep your entire body's health in check, including your mental health. Everyone in your family's gut and brain are very much connected, and when one is off so is the other. Maybe you or your child has experienced this firsthand, like when experiencing a stomachache or feeling really hungry. In these moments, you may recall your brain wasn't performing at its best. So, it makes sense that long-term poor gut health has been linked to some mental illnesses. An out-of-balance gut microbiome (or bacteria) plus accompanying inflammation have been found to cause mental health issues like anxiety and depression.[32] All the more reason to limit added sugar and processed foods and stock up on fresh, whole foods!

CARBOHYDRATES AND OTHER MACRONUTRIENTS

Carbohydrates tend to have a bad reputation, but mostly because there is so much confusing information out there! Carbohydrates are essential macronutrients for children since they are used for active brains and growing muscles. However, problems can arise when carbohydrates are eaten in excess, especially when those carbohydrates are in the form of added sugar or refined carbohydrates.

Not all carbohydrates are created equal. This macronutrient comes in three basic forms: starches, sugars, and fiber. Here's a bit more about each:

- **Starches** are also called *complex carbohydrates* and are low glycemic, meaning they don't cause your blood sugar to spike and drop quickly, a problem that can lead to type 2 diabetes . . . more on this soon! You'll find starches in some vegetables (peas, potatoes, corn), beans and legumes, and grains (oats, rice, wheat, barley, etc.).
- **Sugar** can be naturally occurring, like in fruits and milk, or the added sugars we've been talking about in this chapter. Many of these are high glycemic and will cause your blood sugar to rise quickly then drop just as quickly if consumed alone. Fruit juices, for example, contain more sugar than whole fruit, making juice higher glycemic than fruit.
- **Fiber** is not used as an energy source, but that doesn't mean it is any less important. You'll find fiber in plant foods and it is helpful for digestion, as well as prevention of diseases like type 2 diabetes and heart disease. Fiber takes your body longer to process, which will help you feel full longer between meals, especially when compared to high-glycemic sugars.

Starches and fiber are an essential part of a healthy diet, but sugars (especially added sugars) are not essential. They just taste good! But so do fruits, vegetables, and other nutritious foods.

You may be wondering how carbohydrates can lead to type 2 diabetes. In a nutshell, when you eat carbohydrates, especially sugars or refined carbohydrates, alone this can cause a larger response from insulin. Insulin is the hormone pumped out by your pancreas anytime carbs have entered your body and need to be used as energy or put away for storage. Well, if you are consistently eating large portions of added sugars or refined carbohydrates (think white bread, white rice, pastas that aren't made from whole grains, and sugary cereals) and insulin needs to be released in large amounts over and over again, eventually your pancreas will send out more insulin than is needed. And this can start to happen even when you didn't eat a high-sugar meal. This will eventually lead to cells growing resistant to insulin. Once this happens, type 2 diabetes will not be far behind if diet changes aren't made.

One thing you can do to prevent persistent large blood sugar spikes for you and your kids is to combine carbohydrates with protein every time you eat a meal or snack. The body takes more time to digest protein, and when eaten along with carbohydrates the whole process slows down. This food combining provides more energy and no dramatic spike in blood sugar and insulin. Instead, blood sugar will rise and lower at a steady rate, as it should. Eating fiber at every meal or snack can also help slow digestion and keep blood sugar at a moderate level. The main point here is to eat a variety of foods and not just sugar or high-glycemic carbs in one sitting. Pairing a variety of different healthy macronutrients together can help prevent diet-related health issues.

You and your family can also regulate how often you eat or snack. Eating too often, say every hour, won't allow your organs proper time to rest and reset. If you're eating almost constantly, your pancreas is having to send out insulin almost constantly as well. Eventually, your pancreas will grow tired, and you may find yourself or your family members with a type 2 diabetes diagnosis around the corner.

***

In Japan, it can be difficult for people to have any warning signs of oncoming diabetes. As an expert in diabetes care, Marie thinks this is due to Japanese people not being used to eating sweets and high-glycemic foods, making their bodies more sensitive to sugar. Japanese people also tend to eat less overall compared to Americans. In America, a new type 2 diabetes diagnosis is often accompanied by obesity and other symptoms of metabolic syndrome. But in Japan, onset of type 2 diabetes often does *not* come along with obesity or other diseases. And as more people in Japan eat like Americans do, Marie is seeing more and more people with type 2 diabetes.

Marie's main job as a nutritionist in Japan is to teach the way of low-carbohydrate cooking to people in need, mostly people with type 2 diabetes or who want to start on a low-carb diet. She even cooks this way at home for her dad, who is a diabetic. She's proud of the fact that she can make delicious low-carb meals for him and others in her family. Marie even makes her recipes for *Osechi*, the special Japanese New Year's meal from chapter 6, with no sugar. She instead uses natural sweeteners like monk fruit, stevia, and allulose, and her foods are still tasty!

Not only is Marie helping her dad manage his type 2 diabetes, but she's also teaching others in her family that sugar is often an unneeded ingredient. This is especially true of her nephew. Marie's nephew loves to watch her cook and learn more from her about low-carb recipes and other nutritious foods. He sees that low-carb cooking is something his grandfather needs, but he also sees that anybody can eat this way and reduce lots of sugar from their diet. Marie teaches her nephew to watch out for excess sugar and carbohydrate intake since he has a greater chance of becoming diabetic than many others. She also shares other nutrition knowledge, like how many people take in unnecessary sugar and carbohydrates without intention and that this can get them in trouble with their health. He is always sure to nod and listen well (don't forget, he's a teenager)!

It's Marie's belief that all children have the right to know how and why certain foods can cause potential damage to their body and mind from an early age. Kids learn from experience and from what they see and hear their parents and other adults doing. They're so observant! Unfortunately, many schools in America don't do a great job of teaching basic nutrition to students. This means it's the job of the parents to tell kids all about nutrition, making healthy choices, moving their bodies, and being mindful of how much they eat. It's no secret that most kids love high-sugar sweets and treats, but many parents don't seem to know how much is too much to give to their kids. It's imperative for kids (and everyone else) to have at least basic nutrition knowledge. After all, knowledge is power and when you know how to properly feed yourself, you can empower others around you to do the same.

Marie finds great joy from spending time in the kitchen with her nephew. It's an opportunity for her to share her knowledge through meaningful conversations. And when these conversations are done, they get to eat the delicious dishes they've been making together! Like we've been saying all along, those conversations that happen in and around the kitchen can really have a positive impact on a child's health. Talking with your family about various aspects of food and nutrition may be just the thing you all need to make some changes and start working toward longer, happier, healthier lives.

A FEW EXTRA TIPS

We've been talking quite a bit about type 2 diabetes in this chapter, partly because that is Marie's specialty as a nutritionist and partly because the disease is relatively common. While kids and adults with type 2 diabetes typically require a low-carbohydrate diet, it's important to point out that kids especially need lots of healthy carbs. So, please don't put your child on a low-carbohydrate diet unless recommended by a healthcare professional and for a good reason!

As the body's main source of energy, carbohydrates are a necessary part of all diets. And since growing kids require plenty of energy in the form of calories to develop, learn, and thrive, it's imperative that they eat enough carbohydrates on a daily basis.

With that being said, remember from the previous section that not all carbs are created equal. Your child will get the most nutrition from whole-grain carbohydrate sources. And in case you're wondering, some sources of whole grains include brown rice, oats, quinoa, barley, popcorn (yes, popcorn!), millet, and whole-wheat breads, pastas, and crackers. It's recommended that at least 50% of grain intake for both adults and kids come from whole grains. Of course, the more whole grains you eat, the better. If you and your family are currently only eating enriched grains (like white bread, white rice, etc.), it can be easier than you think to make half of those whole grains instead. Here are some quick tips for eating more whole grains:

- Make at least one meal consist of whole grains per day.
- Swap sugary cereals for whole oats for breakfast (we're not talking about the instant kind of oatmeal!). You can make oatmeal more exciting, tasty, and nutrient-dense by topping it with fruit, nuts, nut butter, or seeds.
- Change your enriched pasta or rice to whole-grain versions. You can also do the same for your sandwich bread, tortillas, rolls, and other products that come in whole-grain versions.
- If you like to meal prep for dinners, use whole grains in your meal prepping recipes.
- Choose whole-grain snacks, like popcorn or whole-wheat crackers—and don't forget to pair these with a little protein for better digestion!

Another popular topic when it comes to carbohydrates is that of gluten-free products. Gluten is a natural protein found in foods like wheat, barley, and rye. These are common ingredients in many carbohydrate foods including breads, pastas, bagels, and cereals. It's also not unheard of to find gluten in soups, baked goods, salad dressings, and some sauces.

Adults and kids with celiac disease, an autoimmune disease, are unable to digest gluten properly, and eating gluten can make them very sick or even damage their intestines. It is also possible to have an allergy or intolerance to gluten. When this is the case, eating gluten can cause some issues like indigestion, trouble with bowel movements, and nausea.

Gluten is found in many whole-grain foods and other healthy carb options. There are many gluten-free products on the market, but many of these are heavily processed and contain lots of ingredients like added sugar and sodium. If you need to be gluten-free, it's best to choose naturally gluten-free carbohydrate sources over processed ones as much as possible. These would include rice, potatoes, squash, legumes, beans, oats, and quinoa, among others. Meats, dairy, fish, and soy are all naturally gluten-free as well.

Finally, it's important to point out that the term *gluten-free* is not synonymous with *low-carb*. A gluten-free diet is one devoid of foods containing gluten but still contains plenty of carbohydrates. A low-carb diet is one that limits all carbohydrates, which forces the dieter to get more calories from protein and fat. Again, a low-carbohydrate diet is mostly necessary for kids and adults with type 2 diabetes and other health issues. It's not a safe option for a healthy, growing kid.

***

If you are a parent who's concerned about your child's health or weight, don't panic. There is no need to take extreme measures with the food you prepare for them. It's important to make just one change to your or your child's diet at a time and continue to take baby steps. Taking things slow will help the whole family gradually get used to eating more nutrient-dense, whole foods while cutting down on calorie-dense foods. If breakfast looks like sugary cereals or pancakes smothered in syrup, lunch looks like strawberry jam and peanut butter sandwiches with chips, snacks look like soda and sweets, dinner looks like pizza, hamburgers, or French fries, and dessert looks like apple pie with ice cream on top, then it may be time for a change. Did you notice that there was lots of added sugar and refined carbs and no vegetables, whole grains, or lean protein in that day of eating?

We've talked about it before, but it's vital for parents to set a good example when it comes to food and nutrition. Setting the example you want your kid to follow can be extremely helpful in him or her becoming healthier. Let your child see that you are also trying to make some positive changes to your life! Children are always watching, and if they see you limiting unnecessary foods and choosing the healthier options instead, they will too. You can all work on prolonging your life together.

So, how can your family start healthy eating? Here are some tips:

- One way to start is by changing what you drink. If you or your child is used to drinking sodas, for example, you could start working on cutting out one soda per day until you're drinking sparkling water instead.

- For breakfast, work on adding fresh fruits, vegetables, and whole grains to your morning. Pair these with an egg or two and maybe last night's leftover chicken you have in your fridge. No one ever said you can't have chicken and veggies for breakfast! There are so many more options than sugary cereals and other refined carbs.

- Don't forget about the bento boxes from chapter 3 for lunch! You'll definitely want to try making your own Japanese rice balls for your and your child's bento boxes. Rice is an unprocessed food with no extra fat or sugar added. And if you eat rice cold, like when you eat rice balls, you may be able to improve your blood sugar. Why? Because rice turns into resistant starch when it is cold. Resistant starches don't get digested and act much like soluble fiber, an important nutrient for gut health. Research shows that eating resistant starches can lead to an improvement in insulin sensitivity, lower blood sugar levels, and a reduced appetite.[33]

- It can be easy to add extra processed snacks to your cart at the grocery store. And once these are in your house, it's hard to avoid them sometimes! Next time, try buying extra fruits, like strawberries or blueberries, that make great snacks instead. Berries are low in carbs and full of antioxidants, and you can eat them with yogurt or sprinkled over salads. Another snack option is to buy various veggies so you can cut them into sticks and eat them with your favorite dips, like the ones found in the recipes below!

- Many people love pasta made from enriched grains. But did you know you can buy different kinds of pasta made from ingredients popular in Japan like edamame (immature soybeans), *shirataki*, or even hearts of palm? *Shirataki* is a very common noodle eaten by Japanese people that is made of devil's tongue, or konjac, a type of yam grown in Japan. Due to its translucent appearance, it's called *shirataki*, Japanese for "white waterfall." Konjac is a low-calorie option, with 97% of it being made from water and the other 3% a type of fiber called glucomannan. *Shirataki* is often eaten in Japan with plenty of vegetables, lean meats, or fish cooked in a big pot in the winter. It is prepared in much the same way as other pastas, cooked with boiling water and eaten with a sauce of your choice.

- Speaking of pasta, it's best to cook pasta "al dente," or to the point of firmness, as this can be better for your body's insulin response. Overcooked pasta becomes soft and loses its form. Interestingly, when this happens soft pasta will release glucose more readily, leading to a larger, quicker rise in blood sugar. When blood sugar rises, insulin is secreted, and too much insulin floating around the body makes it easier for extra fat to be stored.

- If you want to bake cakes or make homemade jelly, monk fruit or stevia is a natural sweetener and a great alternative to sugar. Another option is allulose, which has about one-tenth the calories of table sugar. These sweeteners can be a great way to keep enjoying sweet desserts even when we are trying to make lifestyle changes. But even though desserts made with these alternative sweeteners may have fewer calories, it's still important to watch portions, as it's easy to overeat yummy treats!

HEALTHY KID-FRIENDLY RECIPES

As a nutritionist and recipe developer, Marie enjoys creating delicious dishes that the whole family can enjoy. She comes up with many recipes that are low-carb for her father who has diabetes, and she also often creates gluten-free recipes. As such, Marie has written the healthy recipes below that you can make and eat with your kids.

Low-Carb Creamy Chicken Stew

Here's a gluten-free and low-carb version of a Japanese kids' favorite: creamy stew. This recipe uses almond flour and milk instead of wheat flour and heavy cream. It also includes chicken thighs, another favorite for many kids. Even though it's a healthy option, this stew is still creamy, just the way kids like it! Don't be afraid to add additional vegetables to the recipe, like spinach or avocado. When you switch things up here and there, your kids can enjoy eating different kinds of veggies every time you cook this stew.

Ingredients:

1 pound chicken thighs, cut into bite-size pieces
1/4 teaspoon salt
1/4 teaspoon pepper
5 tablespoons almond flour
6 whole mushrooms
1 whole carrot
3 ounces cauliflower
1 ounce red onion

Any extra veggies you want
2 tablespoons butter
2 cups milk (coconut milk or almond milk is the alternative)
1 cube Maggi bullion
1 bay leaf
Chopped parsley to taste

Instructions:

1. Sprinkle salt and pepper over chicken and let marinate for about 5 minutes. Coat chicken with almond flour.
2. Cut mushrooms into thin pieces. Cut the carrot, cauliflower, red onion, and any extra veggies you choose into bite-size pieces.
3. Place butter in a saucepan and heat over medium-low heat. When the butter is melted, add veggies and chicken to the saucepan and cook over medium-low heat.
4. Pour milk and add a Maggi bullion cube and bay leaf into the saucepan after all the surfaces of the chicken turn brown, and simmer until the liquid gets thicker. Make sure the chicken reaches an internal temperature of at least 165 degrees Fahrenheit.
5. Sprinkle chopped parsley over the dish before serving.

Mini Healthy Hamburger Steaks with Tomato Sauce

Instead of going to a nearby fast-food restaurant, why not cook delicious, nutrient-dense meals with the help of your children in your own home? Yes, you can eat a delicious, healthy hamburger steak at home! Japanese kids are still not used to eating burgers as their regular meals, and they don't even like hamburger buns. If they had to choose, they would pick hamburger steak over American hamburgers every time. Kids love to eat hamburger steaks with one or two veggies like spinach or carrots on the side. In Japan, this dish is simply called "hamburger" and is often made small enough to put into kids' bento boxes.

This low-carb hamburger recipe does not use breadcrumbs for binding the meat. Breadcrumbs are usually used to bind ground meat together when shaping, but since there is no egg in this recipe, we can easily hold the meat together without the crumbs. The recipe also doesn't use ketchup for flavoring. We don't use ketchup since it's usually made with added sugar. Instead, we use chopped tomatoes. Just as onions get sweeter when they get heated up, the acidity of tomatoes becomes milder and sweeter as you cook them. Give it a try!

Ingredients:

1/2 pound ground beef
1/2 pound ground pork
4 ounces chopped onion
1/2 teaspoon nutmeg
1/2 teaspoon garlic powder
1/4 teaspoon salt
1/4 teaspoon pepper
5-6 slices of cheese, cut into 1-inch squares
Coconut oil
6 mushrooms, thinly sliced
6 ounces chopped tomato

Instructions:

1. Add ground beef, ground pork, chopped onions, nutmeg, garlic powder, salt, and pepper to a bowl. Knead well until the texture becomes sticky and ready to be shaped.
2. Divide the meat evenly into 5 or 6 patties and put cheese slices inside each burger as you shape them into an oval.
3. Place coconut oil in a pan and fry the hamburger steaks over medium heat.
4. Add thinly sliced mushrooms to the pan and cook them along with the steaks.
5. Pour finely chopped tomatoes into the pan and simmer until tomatoes lose their solidity.

Homemade Chicken Nuggets

Just like hamburgers, kids like the taste of chicken nuggets. But you can easily make these at home instead of joining the fast-food drive-thru line. Parents are suspicious of what's in chicken nuggets from restaurants, as they should be. Not all chicken nuggets contain just chicken! Chicken nugget contents can be quite different depending on the brand and where you buy them. Unfortunately, some types of nuggets are filled with additives and excess amounts of sodium, and might be deep-fried using old vegetable oils. Chicken quality can also be an issue. If you make your own chicken nuggets at home, you get to buy the chicken and other ingredients you want your children to eat, like free-range chickens or chickens free of antibiotics.

Ingredients:

1 pound ground chicken breast
2 tablespoons mayonnaise
1/4 cup Parmesan cheese
1/2 teaspoon garlic powder
1/4 teaspoon salt
1/4 teaspoon black pepper
1/2 cup almond flour
1 tablespoon coconut oil

Instructions:

1. Add ground chicken, mayonnaise, Parmesan cheese, garlic powder, salt, and pepper to a bowl and mix/knead well.
2. Shape nuggets and then coat each with almond flour.
3. Heat coconut oil in a large frying pan over medium heat and add the chicken nuggets to the pan. Brown on each side and cook until chicken reaches an internal temperature of 165 degrees.
4. Transfer the chicken nuggets to a paper towel–lined plate to cool before eating.

Omelet with Lots of Veggies and Cheese

Eggs are filled with rich nutrients kids need, like protein, choline, and iron. Plus, children can enjoy eating various veggies when put inside a cheesy omelet. Try choosing colorful veggies so kids can enjoy looking at them!

Ingredients:

1 teaspoon Olive oil
4 ounces chopped spinach
4 ounces finely chopped onion
1 red pepper, finely chopped

2 okras, chopped
8 eggs
4 ounces shredded cheese
1/4 teaspoon garlic powder
1/4 teaspoon salt
1/4 teaspoon pepper

Instructions:

1. Put 1 teaspoon of olive oil in a frying pan and heat it over medium heat. Add spinach, onion, red pepper, and okra and sauté until onions turn light brown.
2. Put the sautéed vegetables, eggs, cheese, garlic powder, salt, pepper, and 1 teaspoon of olive oil in a bowl and mix well.
3. Pour the mixture into a large frying pan and cook over medium heat for about 2 minutes
4. Place a lid on the pan and bring the heat down to low. Keep cooking for another 10 minutes.
5. When the surface of the omelet hardens, turn off the heat and transfer to a cutting board so you can cut it into 8 equal pieces.

Low-Carb Dips for Nuggets and Vegetable Sticks

Children will enjoy eating nuggets or vegetable sticks more if they have a few dips to choose from. Compared to the sauces or dips that often come with chicken nuggets from a restaurant or fast-food chain, homemade dips like the ones below have much less added salt, sugar, and other additives. Be sure to read the label before you purchase the product. However, if you're making dips for vegetable sticks, you might need to add a touch more salt and pepper to the recipe so kids can enjoy eating as many veggies as possible. You can also turn any of these recipes into healthy salad dressings by mixing in almond milk, soy milk, or coconut milk to make them more dressing-like. Remember to put these dips on the side of your kids' dishes rather than smothering food with them!

Cheese Dip

1 teaspoon Parmesan cheese
1 teaspoon mayonnaise

1 teaspoon cream cheese
1 tablespoon yogurt

Avocado Dip

1/2 mashed avocado
1/4 teaspoon garlic powder
1 teaspoon mayonnaise
1 teaspoon cream cheese
1 tablespoon yogurt

Sesame Seed Dip

1 teaspoon tahini
1 teaspoon mayonnaise
1 teaspoon cream cheese
1 tablespoon yogurt

Mustard Dip

1 teaspoon mustard
1 teaspoon mayonnaise
1 teaspoon cream cheese
1 tablespoon yogurt

Low-Carb Gluten-Free Garlic Bread

Making homemade bread is easier than you think, especially with this recipe. This gluten-free garlic bread would be a great side on pasta night, or a yummy after-school snack for your kids.

Ingredients:

3 ounces almond flour
3 ounces shredded cheese
3 ounces cream cheese
1 tablespoon Parmesan cheese
1/2 teaspoon garlic powder
1 egg
Pinch of salt

Instructions:

1. Preheat oven to 380 degrees. Prepare a baking sheet with parchment paper.
2. Blend all ingredients until well-mixed.
3. Shaped dough into an oval.
4. Place dough on parchment paper–covered baking sheet.
5. Bake for 10 minutes. Let the bread cool on a wire rack.

***

We hope these recipes inspire you at least a little to try something new. There will be more recipes coming in the following chapter! Remember, one of the most important things you can do is add variety to your family's diet—especially a variety of highly nutritious (and delicious!) foods.

Chapter 8

Advanced Japanese Cooking Tips for a Healthier Life

It's never too late to effect change in your child's life. Sure, the first three years of your little one's life are vitally formative when it comes to their health, but there is still work to do during year four and beyond. Brains are always developing, especially during adolescence. This means there is plenty of time to have a positive impact on your child's nutrition, no matter their age (this means it's not too late for you either!).

HOW TO IMPLEMENT *SHOKUIKU* IN DAILY LIFE

Hopefully by now you understand the overall concept of *Shokuiku* and why the foods Japanese people eat regularly are so nutritious and can aid in living a longer, healthier life. Once you decide to begin eating the *Shokuiku* way, you'll need to know some practical steps to take to get started. The good news is it may be easier than you think to make a few tweaks here and there to your family's diet.

Like with any change you're wanting to make in life, it's best to take small steps at a time to get to where you want you and your family to be. If you try to do a complete 180 overnight, you're almost certainly setting up for failure. The reason so many people "fail" on fad diets is because they make unrealistic and impractical changes quickly and without much thought. But since you are reading this book, you will know how to implement *Shokuiku* in your home in a steady way that will set you up for success.

So, how do you make small, realistic changes? This is done by making one or two changes every few days. For example, if you feel you need to completely rehaul every meal and snack your family eats, start with breakfast. Swap the sugary cereal your kids are eating with whole-grain oats topped with fruit and nuts, or an egg with fresh vegetables. Once breakfast is under control, work on sending your kids to school with a tasty, nutritious bento box. After you and your kids are used to bento boxes, it will be time to work on making more nutrient-dense dinners alongside your kids. And once the three main meals of the day are being eaten the *Shokuiku* way, you can move on to the snacks that are kept in the pantry.

But don't forget one of the most important parts of *Shokuiku*, which is eating at least one meal per day with your family and talking with them about the food, different cultures, nature, and any other topics that will strengthen the family bond. You could work toward making one Japanese meal per week at home, which would be a great opportunity to talk with your family about Japanese culture and everything you've learned in this book. Plus, Japanese meals tend to be very healthy, so doing this would be a win-win!

Making meals more fun for your kids can also help make the transition easier. But don't just fake it until you make it. Be truly enthusiastic about the healthy changes you want your kids to make! It's exciting to improve your health and nutrition, because doing so can greatly impact your life. One way to do this is with the character bento boxes, or *Kyaraben*, from chapter 3. Sending fun messages in your child's school lunchbox is a great way to increase communication between the two of you. They'll surely want to talk to you about the rice ball character you made for them when they get home from school!

But don't just do all of this for your kids. It's important that you and any other adults in the house also practice *Shokuiku*. You can't expect just your kids to be making positive changes to their nutrition if you aren't doing the same. If there is a food you want your kids to eat but you just can't stomach, there are ways around this. Let's say you hate kale but know it is a highly nutritious food that you want your kid to try. You could either come up with an alternative to kale, like spinach, or only give your child kale in their bento box they eat at school. That way, they never have to see you avoiding a food or grimacing at it.

Another idea to help your kids eat more healthy foods the *Shokuiku* way is to turn a food they already like into a healthier version. Like the bun-less hamburgers from the last chapter, you could also make a fish or tofu burger instead of a burger made from cow to help your kids get a wider variety of protein sources. Or you could make the homemade chicken nuggets and dips from the last chapter as well to cut down on your child's added sugar and salt intake. And to avoid creating or nurturing picky eating habits, be sure to only offer your child the food that is on their plate. Once kids are offered too many options, they can quickly become picky.

After a little bit of time and persistence, practicing *Shokuiku* will be second nature to you and your family. Plus, once the health benefits of *Shokuiku* show up (like better energy, more sleep, and lower disease risk) you'll only want more.

ADVANCED JAPANESE COOKING

Part 1: *Dashi*

As we discussed in the previous chapter, Japanese people follow a standard way of preparing dishes called *Ichiju Sansai* (where a meal usually has one soup and three different dishes plus a bowl of rice). Drinking soup at every meal is essential for many Japanese people, and as you can imagine, your stomach gets full pretty fast because of it. In addition to *Ichiju Sansai*, Japanese people tend to watch their portions of food and avoid eating past fullness, or *Hara Hachi Bun Me* (eat until you are 80% full). These two practices on top of all the healthy foods that are customary in Japan help keep the vast majority of the population at a healthy weight.

If you're practicing *Ichiju Sansai* and drinking soup at every meal, it needs to be a light, broth-based soup and not a heavy, cream-based soup. To make things easier, Japanese people created a standard version of a broth-based soup stock called *Dashi* that helps them make many different kinds of soups that are just right for every meal. Think of *Dashi* as chicken or vegetable broths that are commonly used in many American dishes.

Dashi is the stock used not only in Japanese soups but in other boiled dishes. There are two common *Dashi* varieties used for Japanese cooking: *Kombu* (kelp) and *Katsuobushi* (dried smoked bonito flakes). These are used in many authentic Japanese dishes, like *Udon* and *Soba*. Making *Dashi* can take some time, but the payoff in both flavor and health is worth it.

Japanese people tend to use more than one ingredient when making *Dashi*, and there is a specific reason to back this up. But before giving you the reason, let's ask a question. Have you ever heard of the word *umami*? Umami means **a savory** taste and is now considered one of the five flavors our tongues recognize, but that wasn't always the case**.**

The discovery of umami was made by a Japanese professor, Kikunae Ikeda, in 1908, almost 100 years before umami taste receptors were found on the human tongue in 2002.[1] While studying in Germany, Professor Ikeda noticed a unique yet recurring flavor in foods like cheese, tomatoes, and meats that he recognized from *Dashi* back home in Japan. This triggered some additional research by Ikeda and he eventually found that an amino acid, glutamate, was common in all these foods with a savory flavor.[2] Glutamate, or glutamic acid, is the cause of the savory flavor in all umami foods besides the ones already discussed here, like mushrooms, soy sauce, miso, and kimchi. And in case you're wondering, the other four recognized flavors are sweet, sour, salty, and bitter.

So, now is the time to explain why Japanese people tend to mix more than one ingredient when making *Dashi*. It's okay to use just one ingredient like *Konbu* (kelp) when making your *Dashi* since it contains plenty of glutamic acids for your tongue to recognize the umami flavor. But *Dashi* somehow gets tastier when we make it by mixing *Konbu* with other ingredients, like *Katsuobushi* (dried smoked bonito flakes) or shiitake mushrooms. It's more common for Japanese people to use flavor combinations like these when making *Dashi* instead of using just one flavor.

A Japanese scientist, Akira Kuninaka, seems to have all the answers to why people love these specific flavor combinations so much. What he found was that the combination of the glutamic acids in certain foods and nucleotides (such as inosinate or guanylate) in other foods were creating lovely flavors when paired together.[3] It appears that the nucleotides greatly enhance the effect of glutamic acid as well as the intensity of umami being experienced on the tongue.[4] This research means that the two types of *Dashi* Japanese have been using for decades for their everyday meals have been scientifically proven to deliver the best of umami. Japanese people knew they were on to something!

Here is a further breakdown of these two flavor combinations often used to make *Dashi*:

- *Konbu* (kelp) and *Katsuobushi* (dried bonito flakes):
  - *Konbu* contains **glutamic acid.** Other foods containing glutamic acid include cheese, tomatoes, onions, broccoli, miso, and soy sauce.
  - *Katsuobushi* contains **inosine monophosphate,** and so does poultry, beef, and pork.
- *Konbu* (kelp) and shiitake mushrooms:
  - *Konbu* contains **glutamic acid.** Other foods containing glutamic acid include cheese, tomatoes, onions, broccoli, miso, and soy sauce.
  - Shiitake mushrooms contain **guanosine monophosphate,** and so does porcini mushrooms and white mushrooms.

***

Now that you know about *Dashi*, let's look at how to make it as well as a few recipes that incorporate *Dashi*. With some practice, you'll get the hang of making *Dashi*. You can use these *Dashi* recipes in many ways. For example, *Dashi* along with other seasonings, like vinegar and soy sauce, makes a great marinade for vegetables and meats. Japanese people even use *Dashi* for boiling or when simmering veggies to make homemade baby food. Making baby foods this way creates a great opportunity for babies to experience the mild umami taste from early on, without needing to add sugar or salt.

Konbu *and* Katsuobushi Dashi

Ingredients:

2 cups water
2-inch square *Konbu* (kelp)
1 ounce *Katsuobushi* (dried bonito flakes)

Instructions:

1. Put water and *Konbu* in a saucepan and heat on low. If you have extra time, let the *Konbu* soak in the water for about 30 minutes prior to heating.
2. Remove *Konbu* just before water reaches a boil.
3. Add *Katsuobushi* and bring to a simmer for a few minutes.
4. Remove from heat. Strain *Dashi* through a fine strainer into another saucepan or storage container.

Standard Miso Soup Using Konbu *and* Katsuo Dashi *(for 2)*

Ingredients:

5 ounces tofu
1 tablespoon *Wakame* (dried seaweed)
2 cups *Dashi*
3 tablespoons miso

Instructions:

1. Cut tofu into cubes.
2. Add tofu and *Wakame* to *Dashi* in a saucepan and cook over medium heat until it comes to a boil.
3. Turn off heat and dissolve miso into *Dashi.*

Umami Soup with Chicken and Veggies (for 4)

Ingredients:

1 tablespoon olive oil
1 medium tomato, chopped
1 small onion, chopped
3 ounces broccoli, cut into bite-size pieces
5 mushrooms, sliced
1 pound chicken thighs, cut into bite-size pieces
3 cups water
1/2 teaspoon salt
1/2 teaspoon pepper
1/4 cup shredded cheese

Instructions:

1. Put olive oil in a saucepan over medium heat, then add tomatoes, onions, broccoli, mushrooms, and chicken. Sauté until the surface of the chicken changes color.
2. Pour in water. Bring to a simmer and cook until the vegetables become tender. Sprinkle salt, pepper, and cheese on top. Be sure to cook chicken to an internal temperature of 165 degrees Fahrenheit.

Part 2: Fermented Foods

You've probably heard about microbiome (or maybe not), but have you wondered exactly what that is? How about your child's microbiome? There are actually trillions of living bacteria inside your body, mostly inside your gut, both "good" and "bad" bacteria that the gut needs to be in balance to work properly and without issues. These bacteria are responsible for digesting food and keeping bowel movements normal, or not. When your gut microbiome is in good order, you feel better, your digestion is optimal, and your brain works better (your brain and gut are connected, after all).

It's been said that a child's gut microbiome is established over the first few years of their life. But it's fairly easy to change the gut microbiome, both for the better and for the worse. This means it's never too late to improve your and your child's gut health, and you can do this with the help of fermented foods. Fermented foods contain active bacteria that the body can use to restore a gut microbiome that is out of whack, or simply maintain good gut health. Examples of fermented foods include yogurt, sauerkraut, miso, tempeh, kimchi, and kombucha. These foods and others have been linked to not only better gut health but also more diversity of gut microbes, better immunity, and less inflammation.[5]

As you might already know, Japanese people tend to consume a wide variety of fermented foods. This is due in large part to a staple in the country, soy sauce, as well as fermented soybeans called *Natto*. You're probably familiar with soy sauce, but *Natto* is a soybean that has been fermented with the help of a fungus called *Bacillus subtilis*. Because of its strong smell and sticky texture, many people who encounter *Natto* for the first time hesitate to even get close to it. Despite these somewhat off-putting characteristics, many Japanese mothers give *Natto* to their young children. Because of its many health benefits, *Natto* comes highly recommended by nutritionists, like Marie. Kids and adults can greatly benefit from *Natto*'s high content of protein, fiber, and vitamin K.

Another reason fermented foods are popular in Japan dates back to the time before refrigerators. Back then, you could make fermented foods that could be preserved without needing a refrigerator. And because of its distinct seasons and the wide temperature changes from one season to the next, as well as the degree of humidity during the warm summer, Japan has an ideal environment for microorganisms to grow during the food fermentation process.

Soy sauce has become popular all over the world. It can be used not only for Asian cooking but also for everyday cooking. You may already have soy sauce in your kitchen! Soy sauce is made from soybeans, wheat, salt, water, and a fungus called *Koji* (as a side note, if you are gluten-free, a good alternative to soy sauce is wheat-free tamari sauce). When purchasing soy sauce, it's important to choose one that has been naturally brewed or fermented instead of one that has been chemically produced. Naturally brewed soy sauce usually takes at least two months to be fermented, but chemically produced soy sauce is produced within days using hydrolyzed soy protein, corn syrup, and caramel. Be like the Japanese and go for the fermented option! Since soy sauce has glutamic acid in it, you can explore new dimension of umami when using it in your cooking. But keep in mind that a little goes a long way with soy sauce, as it contains extra sodium.

Katsuobushi, mentioned in the *Dashi* section, is also fermented. And you now know that *Katsuobushi* contains inosine monophosphate, which pairs very well with glutamic acid–containing ingredients like soy sauce, providing a maximum umami flavor. Japanese people often put both *Katsuobushi* and soy sauce on top of tofu or boiled vegetables for a simple, healthy, and tasty side dish. You can do this too!

***

Miso is another fermented seasoning unique to Japan that you may have tried before. It is made from salt, *Koji*, and soybeans. Miso has been supporting Japanese people's healthy lifestyles for almost 1,300 years. Because it is fermented, miso contains probiotics that can promote gut health and digestion. It also contains high levels of essential amino acids and potassium, nutrients vital to good health. No wonder Samurais took miso to battle long ago!

For hundreds of years, Japanese people always made their own miso, but these days people seem to be too busy to do the same. The taste of home-made miso can vary from one region to the next based on how much salt or *Koji* is used. The type of *Koji* used also plays a role in the flavor of the final miso product, as there are three types of *Koji*: rice, barely, and soybean.

Marie likes to make miso every year around February and March. She has made delicious miso using organic rice *Koji*, organic black soybeans, and mineral-rich salt from Okinawa. She often shares making homemade miso with her nephew, which is a great *Shokuiku* opportunity for her to share her knowledge with him and for him to learn more about his own culture that he can eventually pass on to his own kids or nephews. However, it usually takes more than 10 months to fully ferment miso and children like her nephew get anxious to taste the miso much sooner!

Fortunately, the process for making miso is not too complicated. The basic steps are:

- Boil soybeans until soft, then smash them.
- Mix the smashed soybeans with salt and *Koji*.
- Make miso balls out of the mixture. The miso balls then need to go into a special plastic bag with an air hole (to prevent molding). Be sure to press hard to get all the air out of the bag.

- Leave the bag in a dark space for at least six months. Leaving it for about 10 months would be best, as the color becomes darker and the taste becomes milder.

It's easy to find recipes and tips online for making your own miso if you want to give it a try (Marie even has a YouTube channel for making miso and other healthy Japanese dishes)! It's fun to watch miso change color over time and start fermenting as the days and weeks go by.

Marie prefers making her own miso at home. This is because, nowadays, anyone can go and buy miso at any supermarket or convenience store in Japan, but it's not the best-quality miso. Since many people these days are too busy to make the *Dashi* needed for homemade miso, they end up buying miso products that already have an umami taste in them. As you already know, miso gets much of its nutritional benefits from the live bacteria and enzymes in it. But most store-bought miso doesn't contain these live enzymes since they eat up all the added umami. Because they want to preserve the umami, manufacturers sterilize miso to remove the beneficial enzymes. If you are going to buy miso, it's best to choose the ones that are unpasteurized, bacteria- and enzyme-rich products that need to be refrigerated. Choosing the right miso, or making your own, will guarantee the best umami flavor!

Miso can be used in other ways besides for making miso soup. And you'll always get that great umami flavor no matter how you use it since miso contains glutamic acid. Marie likes to marinate pork, beef, or chicken in a miso and low-carb sake or mirin (sweet sake) mixture for about an hour to a day in the fridge, depending on how much time she has. Then, once she's ready to grill, sauté, or roast the meats, they're well flavored and have some added nutritional benefits. A good miso with live enzymes will help make the meat extra soft due to the enzymes that start breaking down the protein in the meat into amino acids while it marinates.

It's best to wrap meat up in a paper towel before dipping it into the miso mixture for marinating. That way, there is no miso directly on the meat when you cook it. This may sound odd, but miso gets burnt easily with high heat, so miso-marinated meat should be cooked over low heat (and with a bit of patience). You can marinate vegetables this way, too. Maybe you could make some marinated meat or veggies for your child's next bento box!

You could also use miso instead of tahini or Parmesan cheese in the dip or salad dressing recipes from chapter 7. This would add a lovely umami flavor to your dips and dressings.

One final tip regarding using miso in recipes: To get the nutritional benefits from the live enzymes present in miso, add miso to *Dashi* or any other hot dish near the end of cooking it. Heat can kill the enzymes in miso, so be cautious!

***

Koji can be used in other ways besides as an important ingredient in miso. You can make another marinade, *Shio Koji*, that is similar to miso but takes much less time to ferment. Miso can take up to 10 months to ferment and be ready to eat, but *Shio Koji* can be ready in just 7 to 10 days (or 23 days in the summer)! You may recall that miso requires soybeans to make it, but *Shio Koji* can be made with only rice *Koji*, salt, and water. *Shio Koji* is a great marinade for fish and veggies and may be just the flavor you and your kids need to eat more of these healthy foods. Fish is such a great source of omega-3 fatty acids, protein, and even vitamin D that kids need to grow and develop. Adding just a bit of *Shio Koji* to a fish dish could help turn your child from a seafood hater to a seafood lover.

Here is the recipe for making *Shio Koji*:

Shio Koji

Ingredients:

3.5 ounces (100 g) dried rice *Koji*
1 ounce (30 g) salt
1 1/2 cups (400 ml) water

Instructions:

1. Put *Koji* and salt in a sterilized container and mix well.
2. Pour in water. Mix well.
3. Put a lid on the mixture and leave the container sitting at room temperature for 7 to 10 days.
4. Mix well once a day with a sterilized spoon.
5. When *Shio Koji* become soft and you start to smell sweetness, put it in the refrigerator.

***

You don't always need *Koji* for fermentation. Japanese people love to use a fermentation method called *Asazuke*, which uses only salt and is a relatively quick process that pickles and preserves vegetables for some time. This pickling process is popular in Japan because it helps preserve seasonal veggies in a way that makes them available to eat practically year-round. Another benefit of pickling is that the vegetables are not cooked, and this preserves vitamins, minerals, and other nutrients better than cooking methods that require heat do. Pickling also helps preserve more probiotics for your gut health.

Here is a recipe for sauerkraut, one of the more-famous pickled vegetable foods:

Sauerkraut

Ingredients:

1/2 cabbage (without a stalk)
1 teaspoon salt

Instructions:

1. Shred cabbage into thin pieces, saving one whole cabbage leaf.
2. Put shredded cabbage in a bowl and add salt. Lightly rub salt into cabbage.
3. Put cabbage in a container and place the saved cabbage leaf on top (this prevents the shredded cabbage underneath from hitting the air).
4. Close the container with a lid and leave sitting at room temperature for 2 or 3 days. Let sit for just half a day in the summer.
5. Transfer to the refrigerator and wait until cabbage becomes sour and ready to eat!

Part 3: Tofu

Tofu is a traditional health food in Japan. But besides being packed with nutrition, like plant-based protein and isoflavones, tofu is also versatile (figure 8.1).

Tofu is made from soybeans and is quite economical and easy to cook with (two reasons why it is so popular in Japan). It contains all the essential amino acids, which makes it a complete protein. It's also gentle on the stomach and can be enjoyed by kids and adults, especially when cooked right!

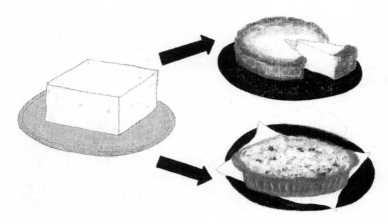

Figure 8.1　Tofu

Eating tofu topped with *Katsuobushi* (dried bonito flakes) and soy sauce is popular in Japan, but you can also use tofu to make hamburgers (or rather, tofu burgers). Or, you can try Marie's tofu casserole (or "gratin") recipe that is meant to be eaten out of small, individual casserole plates. These small casseroles can help you and your family eat a well-portioned meal the *Shokuiku* way.

Tofu Gratin Casserole

Ingredients:

10 ounces tofu
2 ounces tuna (from a can)
1 tablespoon miso
1/4 teaspoon garlic powder
1 tablespoon olive oil
2 ounces spinach
Pinch of salt
2 ounces shredded cheese

Instructions:

1. Wrap tofu in a paper towel and put a weight over it to drain the water. Leave to drain for 1 to 2 hours.

2. Put tofu, tuna, miso, and garlic powder in a bowl and mix until smooth.
3. Add olive oil to a frying pan, then add spinach and a pinch of salt and cook over medium heat.
4. Add the tofu mixture to the frying pan and continue cooking until there is no more liquid in the pan.
5. Transfer the mixture to a small casserole dish and sprinkle cheese over it.
6. Bake for 15 minutes at 300 degrees, or until the cheese is a nice brown color.

Kids (and many adults) love desserts. As a parent, you may be wondering how you can make sweets and treats healthier for your child. The next recipe for tofu cheesecake is an excellent dessert choice, as you can reduce calorie intake by adding protein-rich tofu. You can feel good about making this high-protein tofu cheesecake that also happens to be extra smooth and tasty!

Tofu Cheesecake

Ingredients:

7 ounces tofu
1 ounce butter
8 ounces cream cheese
3 ounces allulose (substitute for sugar)
2 eggs
3 drops vanilla oil

Instructions:

1. Drain tofu a day before making the cheesecake. Butter and cream cheese need to be room temperature by the time you start.
2. Place tofu, butter, and cream cheese in a bowl. Mix well.
3. Add allulose, eggs, and vanilla oil. Mix well.
4. Add mixture to a cake tin (6 inches in diameter) that has been lined with parchment paper.
5. Bake at 300 degrees for 1 hour.

Chapter 9

Shinto Culture

Incorporating spirituality into eating is key to having lifelong respect and adoration for food and what it does for your body. Regardless of your religion, you can (and you can help your children) adopt a more meaningful, healthier relationship with food. In fact, you don't need religion at all to do this!

Much of Japanese culture stems from something called Shintoism. And though Shintoism may sound like a religion, it's more accurately described as a Japanese way of life. Shintoism is culture in Japan. Early beliefs and aspects of Shintoism have shaped much of the culture of Japan you see today. Shintoism is a beautiful, spiritual celebration of life and can be seen practically everywhere: food, the arts, politics, family life, and even sports.[1] The roots of Shintoism date back as far as 1000 BCE, and followers believe the nature around them is full of spiritual powers or gods called *Kami*.[2] The estimated 87 million followers of Shintoism in Japan regularly pay homage to these gods that are believed to live in animals, plants, mountains, air, rivers, lakes, people, and other aspects of the natural world.[3]

In Shintoism, there are thousands of *Kami*. There is a *Kami* of the sea, the rivers, the mountains, the sun, and more.[4] When visiting a Shinto shrine (figure 9.1), followers offer Japanese staples like rice, fish, and vegetables to the *Kami* as a way to show respect and gratitude for what has been provided from nature to the prayerful. When food is offered while praying to gods, it's like having a meal with the gods with the hope that feelings and wishes will be better heard. People see fresh foods like fish and vegetables they get from Japan's backyard as blessings, which is why they show so much gratitude toward nature.[5] This appreciation takes place not only in Shinto shrines but also at home and even at work. Basically, the Japanese and especially

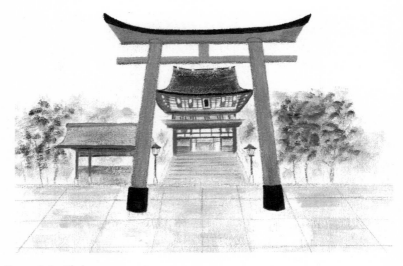

Figure 9.1   Shrine

those who follow Shintoism are consistently grateful for their food. And this gratefulness leads to a spiritual connection to food, something that may sound far-fetched to many Americans.

Japanese people feel they need help from all the different *Kami* to live a healthy, long life. And this may be because of some of the earliest roots of Shintoism. Marie likes to recount the origins of the *Kami* of fire. Japanese people used to live in homes where the fireplace was built into the center of the main living space. Families would do everything around this fire—cook, eat, get warm, sleep. The people of Japan back then couldn't survive without the help of the fire, and they saw the fire as a god. After all, you can't cook without fire, and back then you couldn't get warm without it either. Japanese people also started viewing food as a *Kami* and would offer food to the other gods who were helping them live.

We tend to forget that humans cannot live without nature. As a country surrounded by mountains and the sea, it's almost impossible not to be in awe of the beauty of Japan. But beyond this beauty is the fact that much of the country's resources, including food, comes from within its borders. Because of Shintoism's deep respect for the food that comes from nature, food is also a symbol of spirituality.[6] This spiritual connection to food is the reason why so many Japanese people opt for fresh, whole foods and seasonal fruits and vegetables.

Even the popularity of fish in the country has roots in Shintoism. Early laws of Shintoism prohibited eating meat because it was seen as unclean. However, other protein foods like fish, tofu, and those from plants were fair game,[7] and these still make up much of the diet in Japan today. The Shinto focus on purity is applied to food in other ways too. For example, many Japanese people prefer eating natural, whole foods over unnatural or processed food, like choosing to eat a fresh tomato instead of factory-made ketchup.

Besides all these crossovers between food and nature, food is also seen as a reflection of the Japanese person who eats it.[8] The aspect of purity in Shintoism serves as a bit of motivation for its followers to organize their dinner plates in a clean fashion. Not taking the time to enjoy your food or eating in any way that is unhealthy (whether it be the actual food or how the food is eaten) can be equated to a person not paying attention to their own health or the state of their body.[9]

As you can hopefully see by now, many aspects of eating the *Shokuiku* way can be linked to Shintoism. We've been talking about everything from making bento boxes to having more mealtime conversations with your family to learning about seasonal vegetables. And, of course, the importance of showing gratitude for your food. All these parts of *Shokuiku* are, in fact, spiritual. It's funny, then, that both Marie and Motoko will tell you that when you ask a Japanese person if they are Shinto, they will almost always say no. However, all Japanese people exercise Shinto culture constantly—they just don't realize it, as it's no longer a conscious effort. Because Shintoism has become synonymous with Japanese culture, the people there think they are simply following their cultural roots when in reality they're following Shinto roots! Regardless of where these customs started, the fact remains that spirituality is an important part of life, including food.

BUT FIRST, WHAT IS SPIRITUALITY?

We realize that spirituality can be difficult to grasp for some people, especially if you don't consider yourself to be a spiritual person. So, with that in mind, it seems important to define the term a bit here before we move on.

Your relationship with spirituality can look completely different from that of your friends and family, even the person that sleeps next to you! Spirituality can be religious, but it doesn't have to be. It basically means you have a connection with something greater than yourself, and that could be the gods, the earth, the ocean, the trees, the sky, or many other things.

Being spiritual may even help you find more purpose and meaning in life, restore hope, and find a sense of community.[10]

Spirituality often gives people a sense of being alive and interconnected to others and the world around them.[11] In Japan, those who practice Shintoism recognize that both society and nature are interconnected. This leads to embracing harmony in the world around them.

Being spiritual can offer a source of comfort we so often need. And, you can find this type of comfort and gratitude from preparing and enjoying meals with your family, having meaningful conversations around the kitchen table, and starting a garden in your backyard. You will experience deeper, more spiritual connections with your family members from sharing gratitude for your meals together.

SPECIAL EVENTS IN SHINTO CULTURE

Cultural events happen year-round in Japan. In fact, there seems to be at least one every month. Many of these involve food as well as aspects of Shintoism. You may even see advertisements for upcoming Shinto holidays and events in supermarkets, with special foods being marketed for the days. These cultural events are so important in Japan that they are celebrated not only in families' homes but also in schools. The kids love these special days, as they get to share them with both their families and their friends at school. Plus, the school nutritionists make their school lunches more exciting by using colors and foods to commemorate the events.

Introducing a few of these events may help you better understand the connections between the people of Japan, its culture, and, of course, food.

The biggest event of the year in Japan is New Year's Day. You already learned about *Osechi*, or the New Year's Day meal in Japan that carries lots of meaning and well-wishes for the new year. But the festivities go beyond *Osechi*.

There are many rituals that occur around New Year's Day in Japan. Even though some Japanese families celebrate the new year in traditional ways, others take a more casual route. In Japan, the days surrounding the new year are meant for praising and thanking the gods for all that was provided in the preceding year, and praying for more prosperity, health, and happiness in the year to come. The whole family comes together for the new year to be thankful for the bounty provided by nature.

It's customary for Japanese families to do a bit of a deep clean, or *Oosouji*, of their home as a way to start the new year on a clean slate. But they don't do this on January 1, since this day is solely for eating, resting, and celebrating. Everything about the new year in Japan is about, well, newness. Many kids wake up on New Year's Day with new clothes to wear. There is also a tradition called *Otoshidama* where kids receive money in envelopes from their parents and grandparents. Japanese children really have a great day on January 1—there are special games for them to play, and almost anything goes in terms of fun for them on this day and they won't get in trouble!

There's plenty for the adults to do on New Year's Day and the days surrounding it as well. Some may go out to buy *Fukubukuro*, or "grab bags" containing a mix of random items sold at a discounted price. And although the adults may spend hours and hours preparing *Osechi* leading up to New Year's Day (with a bit of help from the kids, of course), once the day arrives, they simply sit back, relax, eat, drink, and be merry. Families enjoy wonderful conversations and opportunities for bonding while preparing special foods for *Osechi*. Family recipes are handed down from one generation to the next, and the elders offer their wisdom to their children and grandchildren.

Hatsumode is an important spiritual event surrounding New Year's Day. It is a tradition in which large crowds of people visit Shinto shrines on the 1st, 2nd, or 3rd of January. While at the shrine, Japanese people will thank the gods for the previous year and pray for another year of health and happiness. Some of these shrines have festivals at the start of the new year that include food stands, plenty of prayer, and new lucky charms for sale (it's customary to throw out the previous year's charms when buying new ones).[12]

People can partake in *Hatsumode* at any shrine they choose. Some prefer to go to their local shrine, while others like to go to the most popular Shinto shrines with the largest crowds. Some shrines have fun games like *Omikuji*, a simple fortune-telling activity that will tell you how lucky you'll be in the new year. But you have to be a little brave to play this game, because if you draw *daikyo* that means you will have the worst luck in the new year![13]

There are many Japanese New Year's Day traditions, and the majority of them involve food. From December 31 to January 7, special foods are eaten in Japan.

On New Year's Eve, families eat soba together and mostly stay home—a very different scene from the traditional New Year's Eve in America! Soba are noodles made from buckwheat, and Japanese people have been eating them since the 13th and 14th centuries when rulers would give the hungry soba noodles as a blessing.[14] These days, the soba noodles symbolize many things. First, they symbolize resilience because buckwheat plants are able to withstand harsh conditions while they grow. The long noodles also represent longevity to those who eat them. And, because soba noodles are very easy to bite through, eating them on New Year's Eve signifies chopping off the old year.[15]

Once New Year's Day arrives, it's time to eat *Osechi*, the meal that took many hours to cook, prepare, and assemble in *Jubako*. Since we already talked about the foods of *Osechi* quite a bit in chapter 6, we'll just introduce a couple more here. One of these is *Kagami Mochi*, or "mirror rice cake." This creation consists of two or three rice cakes stacked on top of each other, with a bitter orange adorning the very top. The *Kagami Mochi* may be displayed in the family home on a small altar on a sheet (called a *Shihobeni*) that is thought to have the power to ward off any house fires in the coming year.[16] It's actually displayed for a week or two before it is eaten by the family. Eating the mirror rice cake is called *Kagami Biraki*, or "mirror opening," and eating it with loved ones is meant to give luck to the family in the new year.[17]

Another *Osechi* food is *Zoni*, or mochi rice cake soup. The soup got its start with the samurai and was made to give the fighters strength. In the 1400s, Japanese people started offering mochi (rice cakes) to gods on New Year's Eve. Because of this offering, and because the mochi was already prepared, there would be ingredients to easily make *Zoni* the next day, or New Year's Day. *Zoni* is believed to bring the soup drinker a successful new year.[18]

Because so many foods are made for *Osechi*, families have leftovers for days. But that all stops on January 7, because on the 7th Japanese families eat *Nanakusa Gayu*. This dish that translates to "seven herbs rice porridge" symbolizes health and warding off evil in the new year. It's a healthy and light meal that feels good to eat after six days of indulgence.

***

Besides New Year's Day, there are many other events rooted in Shintoism throughout the year in Japan. Here are a few of them:

Okuihajime: A fun and sweet tradition marking a baby's 100th day of life, *Okuihajime* is a delight. The word *Okuihajime* translates to "first meal." The ritual is set up by the baby's parents, and friends and family attend to watch the bundle of joy partake. This first meal is set up in the same way as most Japanese meals are, with one soup and three dishes (or *Ichiju*

Sansai from chapter 7). The meal usually contains cooked rice, fish, soup, and plenty of fresh vegetables. Now, you may be asking yourself how a 100-day-old baby is going to eat all this food. The answer is, he's not! The tradition is a mixture of a cute photo op and a way for the eldest member of the family to wish the baby a long, happy, healthy life.[19] This family member even pretends to feed the baby the food three times in a specific order of rice, soup, rice, fish, rice, soup.[20] Before the ritual ends, the eldest family member will touch chopsticks that have previously touched a stone at a shrine to the baby's gums to wish for a healthy set of teeth.[21]

Shichi-go-san: Every year on November 15, three-year-old girls, five-year-old boys, and seven-year-old girls go with their families to shrines to pray for a healthy life. The ages may sound random to you, but they have meaning in Japan that dates back many hundreds of years. In Japan, once a child reaches three years old they are allowed to grow out their hair; at five, boys are now old enough to wear trousers (or *hakama*) with their kimonos; and at seven, girls tie their first *obi*, or sash.[22] On this eventful day at the shrine, all members of the family dress up, with many of the children wearing traditional kimonos (figure 9.2). Besides their special outfits and prayers, the children being honored during *Shichi-go-san* also carry bags decorated with pictures of nature that contain a long, thin candy called *chitose ame*.[23] The candy represents long life due to its stretched look.[24] Because kimonos are tight, many children don't like wearing them for long, including Motoko's son. However, she was able to get him to wear a kimono during *Shichi-go-san* with a little old-fashioned bribery that included *chitose ame*. The cute pictures of her son made the bribe very much worth it!

Setsubun: On the last day of winter (according to the Japanese lunar calendar) many families come together to partake in a tradition called *Setsubun*. One of the main events of the day entails ridding the house of demons, or *oni*, and there are a couple different ways to do this. In some families, the head of the household throws roasted soybeans held in a wooden box out the front door while yelling "*Oni wa soto! Fuku wa uchi!*" or "Demons get out! Good luck come in!"[25] But in some other families, the father dresses up like a demon while the children throw soybeans at him and yell these same words (figure 9.3). The kids love it (although some of the smaller ones get scared of the *oni*)! These rituals are meant to purify the family home of any misfortune sticking around from the previous year.[26] Family members also eat one roasted soybean for each year of their life during *Setsubun*. This is done to wish for good luck in the new year, as soybeans are a symbol of luck in Japanese culture.

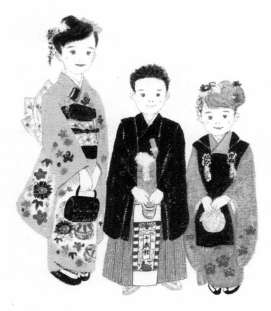

Figure 9.2   Shichi-go-san

Hina-matsuri: The tradition of *Hina-matsuri*, or Japanese Girls' Day, takes
  place annually on March 3 as a way to pray for health for young Japanese girls (figure 9.4). *Hina-matsuri* is celebrated using special dolls and
  food. During this day, families of young girls display sets of *hina* dolls
  that were either bought when their daughter was born or passed down
  through generations.[27] *Hina* dolls date all the way back to the Hein period
  about 1,250 years ago. Marie has fond memories of looking at her *hina*
  dolls and remembers the day being very exciting. Marie's *hina* dolls were
  very old when she was a young girl and her mother still has them to this
  day! The dolls are only displayed on *Hina-matsuri*, as displaying them
  on other days could mean bad luck. Traditional foods are prepared and
  eaten on Japanese Girls' Day as well, with rice wine and rice cakes being
  displayed along with the *hina* dolls.[28] But there is plenty of food for eating as well! Family members will cook delicious savory foods and even
  some sweets to commemorate the day. This day is just one more example
  of how Japanese families blend culture with food to show appreciation.
Kodomo-no-hi: After Japanese Girls' Day comes Children's Day (although
  some refer to it as Boys' Day). On May 5 of every year, homes of young

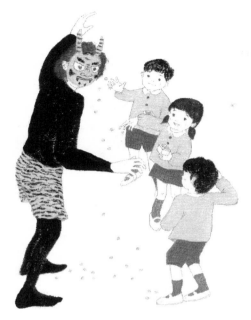

Figure 9.3   Setsubun

boys will display colorful carp fish flags outside. In Japan, carp are viewed as mighty fish that can transform into dragons.[29] Traditionally, all family members get a carp of a different color displayed outside their home, with any little boys living in the house being represented by a bright blue carp flag. Samurai armor is also used to decorate the homes of little boys to help wish for strong, powerful boys.[30] Motoko's parents bought a lovely armor set for her son, so lovely, in fact, that he thought the armor was real! But that's not all that happens on *Kodomo-no-hi*. There must be food! Special dishes are made for this day, like *chimaki*, which is a sticky rice cake containing savory flavors like pork, shrimp, and shiitake mushrooms.[31]

We've shared these Japanese events to help you see how food can be spiritual. As you probably noticed, all these traditions involve food in one way or another. These traditions also all involve families spending time together, eating together, and bonding. What could be better than that?

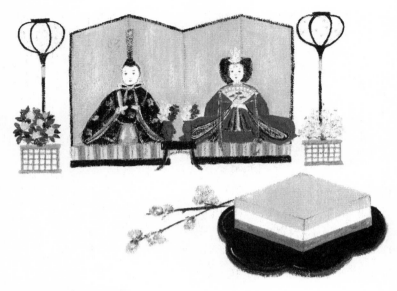

Figure 9.4   Hinamatsuri

HOW SHINTOISM AND *SHOKUIKU* INTERSECT

In America, many people tend to eat meals on the go or while staring at a device. When a person eats in this way it's easy to argue that they're not paying attention to their bodies or their health. And definitely not their spirituality! You would be hard-pressed to find an American who views food as a spiritual symbol—we're not saying they don't exist, but it's not a common practice. Whether your family is spiritual or not, aspects of Shintoism can still be applied when practicing *Shokuiku.* The two mesh well!

Aside from *Shokuiku*, you've actually been learning many things about Shintoism for many chapters now as well. As an example, let's look at talking with your family about where the food you are all about to eat comes from. These discussions may include things like the farmer who grew the food, or how water and the sun were necessary to nourish the food, or even how the food was picked at the point of ripeness. You may not realize it, but these are spiritual conversations. They're spiritual conversations because you and your family are talking about how the foods before you were grown by the elements and then picked from the earth. This shows an interconnectedness to the earth and even other people you've never met, like the farmer who grew your beans.

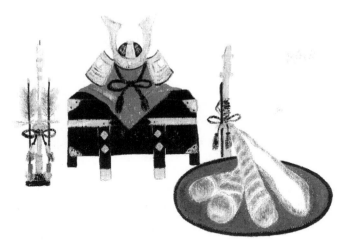

Figure 9.5 Kodomo-no-hi

Spirituality toward food can look different to many people. There are tons of ways to be spiritual since there are no set rules to follow. After all, spirituality isn't religion. Both you and your children can be spiritual as you teach them the value of how eating living things like plants and animals gives you all literal life. And you can learn alongside your kids as you teach them that nature both *is* precious life and *gives* precious life.

Your family can be spiritual toward food by remembering a few Japanese terms:

- *Ikasarete-iru* means showing deeper gratitude toward a food source. It's showing a sincere appreciation for many people's hard work to cultivate the food as well as the power of the sun, rain, soil, and even micro-organisms to bring your family the meals before them. Instead of saying "I live because I can eat rice," *Ikasarete-iru* would be roughly translated to "I'm allowed to live because of eating rice and it is a blessing that I must be thankful for."[32] Basically, food gives you literal life.
- *Mottainai* means to appreciate what you have, including what you eat (and every single ingredient). When your family understands and appreciates where food comes from, you will naturally start thinking about how food affects you all. This will lead to cooking no more than what is needed. Reduce, recycle, and don't throw away!
- *Itadakimasu* is a tradition you've heard about before (in chapter 6 to be exact). It's rooted in Shintoism and shows appreciation for food, but any

religion or culture can practice it. Families join hands (much like other cultures "say grace") before a meal and say "*Itadakimasu*," which means "I partake / I will have." This tradition can help your family see that we are all intertwined and should show gratitude for all the efforts of the earth and the people that come together to bring nourishing meals to the table.

There are many ways to be spiritual. And one of these ways is to see food as a spiritual symbol as they do in Shintoism. Embarking on your *Shokuiku* journey with your family is the perfect time to work on spirituality. The spiritual practices that join food and your family don't need to be conscious efforts, as spirituality is rooted in many aspects of *Shokuiku*. As you and your children practice *Shokuiku*, all will naturally become more spiritual beings!

Notes

CHAPTER 1

1. Ana Swanson, "The U.S. Isn't the Fattest Country in the World, but It's Close," *Washington Post*, April 22, 2015, https://www.washingtonpost.com/news/wonk/wp/2015/04/22/youll-never-guess-the-worlds-fattest-country-and-no-its-not-the-u-s.

2. Lise Eliot, PhD, *What's Going On in There?* (New York: Bantam Books, 2000), 425.

CHAPTER 2

1. "Japan Shows Food Education Works," Medium, July 7, 2017, https://medium.com/@BCFN_Foundation/japan-shows-food-education-works-6b7aa32cb809.

2. "Average Life Expectancy in Selected Countries as of 2020," Statista, October 28, 2021, https://www.statista.com/statistics/236583/global-life-expectancy-by-country.

3. Aleksandra Malachowska and Marzena Jezewska-Zychowicz, "Does Examining the Childhood Food Experiences Help to Better Understand Food Choices in Adulthood?" *Nutrients* 13, no. 3 (2021): 983, https://www.mdpi.com/2072-6643/13/3/983/htm.

4. "Nutrition and Early Brain Development," Urban Child Institute, March 25, 2011, http://www.urbanchildinstitute.org/articles/updates/nutrition-and-early-brain-development.

5. Jill Stamm, PhD, *Bright from the Start* (New York: Avery, 2007), 12.

6. Stamm, *Bright from the Start*, 15.

7. Lise Eliot, PhD, *What's Going On in There?* (New York: Bantam Books, 2000), 425.

8. "Child Development and Early Learning," UNICEF, *Facts for Life*, 4th ed. (2010), https://factsforlife.org/03/index.html.

9. T. Momose, J. Nishikawa, T. Watanabe, Y. Sasaki, M. Senda, K. Kubota, Y. Sato, M. Funakoshi, and S. Minakuchi, "Effect of Mastication on Regional Cerebral Blood Flow in Humans Examined by Positron-Emission Tomography with O-labelled Water and Magnetic Resonance Imaging," *Archives of Oral Biology* 42, no. 1 (January 1997): 57–61, https://pubmed.ncbi.nlm.nih.gov/9134116.

10. "Breastfeeding: Data & Statistics," Centers for Disease Control and Prevention, 2021, https://www.cdc.gov/breastfeeding/data/facts.html.

11. Rita Robinson, "DHA—The Experts Say It's Essential," NY Metro Parents, August 21, 2001, https://www.nymetroparents.com/article/DHA-the-experts-say-it-s-essential20110418.

12. "Nutrition—When, What and How to Introduce Solid Foods," Centers for Disease Control and Prevention, 2021,

13. E. Mok, C. A. Vanstone, S. Gallo, P. Li, E. Constantin, and H. A. Weiler, "Diet Diversity, Growth and Adiposity in Healthy Breastfed Infants Fed Homemade Complementary Foods," *International Journal of Obesity* 41 (2017): 776–82, https://www.nature.com/articles/ijo201737.

14. J. Liu, Y. Cui, L. Li, L. Wu, A. Hanlon, J. Pinto-Martin, A. Raine, and J. R. Hibbeln, "The Mediating Role of Sleep in the Fish Consumption—Cognitive Functioning Relationship: A Cohort Study," *Scientific Reports* 7, 17961 (2017), https://doi.org/10.1038/s41598-017-17520-w.

CHAPTER 3

1. Jill Stamm, PhD, *Bright from the Start* (New York: Avery, 2007), 13.

2. John Asano, "A Brief History of Bento," All about Japan, October 15, 2015, https://allabout-japan.com/en/article/300.

3. Sheila M. Innis, "Dietary Fatty Acids and Brain Development," *Journal of Nutrition* 137, no. 4 (April 2007), http://jn.nutrition.org/content/137/4/855.long.

4. Edward F. Zigler, Matia Finn-Stevenson, and Nancy W. Hall, *The First Three Years and Beyond* (New Haven: Yale University Press, 2002), 176.

CHAPTER 4

1. C. A. Forestell, "Flavor Perception and Preference Development in Human Infants," *Annals of Nutrition & Metabolism* 70, supp. 3 (2017): 17–25, https://pubmed.ncbi.nlm.nih.gov/28903110.

2. Michael Frederick and Gordon Gallup, "The Demise of Dinosaurs and Learned Taste Aversions: The Biotic Revenge Hypothesis, *Ideas in Ecology and Evolution* 10, no. 1 (2017): 47–54, https://ojs.library.queensu.ca/index.php/IEE/article/view/6802.

3. M. Profet, "Pregnancy Sickness as Adaptation: A Deterrent to Maternal Ingestion of Teratogens," in *The Adapted Mind: Evolutionary Psychology and the Generation of Culture*, ed. J. H. Barkow, L. Cosmides, and J. Tooby (Oxford: Oxford University Press, 1992), 327–65.

4. Lise Eliot, PhD, *What's Going On in There?* (New York: Bantam Books, 2000), 180.

5. Yi Hui Liu, MD-MPH, and Martin T. Stein, MD, "Feeding Behaviour of Infants and Young Children and Its Impact on Child Psychosocial and Emotional Development," in *Encyclopedia on Early Childhood Development*, 2nd ed. (September 2013), 11, https://www.child-encyclopedia.com/pdf/expert/child-nutrition/according-experts/feeding-behaviour-infants-and-young-children-and-its-impact-child.

6. Eliot, *What's Going On?*, 193.

7. Nancy Butte, PhD, RD, Kathleen Cobb, MS, RD, Johanna Dwyer, DSc, RD, Laura Graney, MS, RD, William Heird, MD, Karyl Rickard, PhD, RD, "The Start Healthy Feeding Guidelines for Infants and Toddlers," in the Journal of the Academy of Nutrition and Dietetics, 104, 3 (March 2004): 442–454, https://www.jandonline.org/article/S0002-8223(04)00084-7/fulltext.

8. "Feeding a Picky Eater: Do's and Don'ts," Children's Hospital of Philadelphia, October 31, 2019, https://www.chop.edu/news/dos-and-donts-feeding-picky-eaters.

9. Jennifer S. Savage, Jennifer Orlet Fisher, and Leann L. Birch, "Parental Influence on Eating Behavior," *Journal of Law, Medicine & Ethics* 35, no. 1 (2007): 22–34, https://www.ncbi.nlm.nih.gov/pmc/articles/PMC2531152.

10. Butte et al., "The Start Healthy Feeding Guidelines for Infants and Toddlers."

CHAPTER 5

1. C. Bernard Gesch, Sean M. Hammond, Sarah E. Hampson, and Anita Eves, "Influence of Supplementary Vitamins, Minerals and Essential Fatty Acids on the Antisocial Behaviour of Young Adult Prisoners," *British Journal of Psychiatry* 181 (July 2002): 22–28.

2. "Japan Shows Food Education Works," Barilla Center for Food and Nutrition, July 7, 2007, https://www.barillacfn.com/en/magazine/food-and-society/japan-shows-food-education-works.

3. "The National School Lunch Program," United States Department of Agriculture, November 2017, https://fns-prod.azureedge.us/sites/default/files/resource-files/NSLPFactSheet.pdf.

4. "National School Lunch Program Meal Pattern Chart," United States Department of Agriculture, September 9, 2019, https://www.fns.usda.gov/nslp/national-school-lunch-program-meal-pattern-chart.

5. Katie Adolphus, Clare Lawton, and Louis Dye, "The Effects of Breakfast on Behavior and Academic Performance in Children and Adolescents," *Frontiers in Human Neuroscience* 7 (2013): 425, https://www.ncbi.nlm.nih.gov/pmc/articles/PMC3737458.

6. Adolphus, Lawton, and Dye, "The Effects of Breakfast on Behavior and Academic Performance in Children and Adolescents."

7. David Benton, Alys Maconie, and Claire Williams, "The Influence of the Glycaemic Load of Breakfast on the Behaviour of Children in School," *Physiology & Behavior* 92, no. 4 (November 2007): 717–24, https://pubmed.ncbi.nlm.nih.gov/17617427.

8. Benton, Maconie, and Williams, "The Influence of the Glycaemic Load of Breakfast on the Behaviour of Children in School."

9. Caroline Taylor and Pauline Emmett, "Picky Eating in Children: Causes and Consequences," *Proceedings of the Nutrition Society* 78, no. 2 (May 2019): 161–69, https://pubmed.ncbi.nlm.nih.gov/30392488.

10. Taylor and Emmett, "Picky Eating in Children: Causes and Consequences."

11. "What Is ADHD?" American Psychiatric Association, July 2017, https://www.psychiatry.org/patients-families/adhd/what-is-adhd.

12. "What Is ADHD?" American Psychiatric Association.

13. Kimberly Holland and Elsbeth Riley, "ADHD by the Numbers: Facts, Statistics and You," Healthline, April 13, 2018.

14. Holland and Riley, "ADHD by the Numbers: Facts, Statistics and You."

15. R. Schnoll, D. Burshteyn, and J. Cea-Aravena, "Nutrition in the Treatment of Attention-Deficit Hyperactivity Disorder: A Neglected but Important Aspect," *Applied Psychophysiological Biofeedback* 28, no. 1 (March 2003): 63–75, https://pubmed.ncbi.nlm.nih.gov/12737097.

16. Jill Stamm, PhD, *Bright from the Start* (New York: Avery, 2007), 14.

17. Michelle Roberts, "Experts Say Food May Contribute to Anger, Violent Behavior," CBS News Boston, March 15, 2013, http://boston.cbslocal.com/2013/03/15/experts-say-food-may-contribute-to-anger-violent-behavior.

18. John Bohannon, "The Theory? Diet Causes Violence. The Lab? Prison," *Science* 325, no. 5948 (September 25, 2009): 1614–16, http://science.sciencemag.org/content/325/5948/1614.full?sid=f17a8d10-851c-4e03-96c0-3f11e729bbe8.

19. Gesch, Hammond, Hampson, and Eves, "Influence of Supplementary Vitamins."

20. Schnoll, Burshteyn, and Cea-Aravena, "Nutrition in the Treatment."

21. Schnoll, Burshteyn, and Cea-Aravena, "Nutrition in the Treatment."

22. Lise Eliot, PhD, *What's Going On in There?* (New York: Bantam Books, 2000), 195.

CHAPTER 6

1. Alan L. Sroufe, "Early Relationships and the Development of Children," *Infant Mental Health Journal* 21 (2002): 67–74.

2. "Average Child Gets $6,500 Worth of Toys in Their Lifetime," SWNS Digital, November 16, 2016, http://www.swnsdigital.com/2016/11/average-child -gets-6500-worth-of-toys-in-their-lifetime.

3. Edward F. Zigler, Matia Finn-Stevenson, and Nancy W. Hall, *The First Three Years and Beyond* (New Haven: Yale University Press, 2002), 174; A. Chavez, C. Martinez, and T. Yaschine, "Nutrition, Behavioral Development and Mother-Child Interaction in Young Rural Children, *Federation Proceedings* 334, no. 7 (1975): 1574–82.

4. Edward F. Zigler, Matia Finn-Stevenson, and Nancy W. Hall, *The First Three Years and Beyond* (New Haven: Yale University Press, 2002), 174; A. Chavez, C. Martinez, and T. Yaschine, "Nutrition, Behavioral Development and Mother-Child Interaction in Young Rural Children, *Federation Proceedings* 334, no. 7 (1975): 1574–82.

5. Ryan Dwyer, Kostadin Kushlev, and Elizabeth Dunn, "Smartphone Use Undermines Enjoyment of Face-to-Face Social Interactions," *Journal of Experimental Social Psychology* 78 (September 2018); 233–39.

6. L. Alan Sroufe, "Early Relationships and the Development of Children."

7. Yi Hui Liu, MD-MPH, and Martin T. Stein, MD, "Feeding Behaviour of Infants and Young Children and Its Impact on Child Psychosocial and Emotional Development," in *Encyclopedia on Early Childhood Development*, 2nd ed. (September 2013), 11–15, https://www.child-encyclopedia.com/pdf/expert/child -nutrition/according-experts/feeding-behaviour-infants-and-young-children-and-its -impact-child.

CHAPTER 7

1. Ana Swanson, "The U.S. Isn't the Fattest Country in the World, but It's Close," *Washington Post*, April 22, 2015, https://www.washingtonpost.com/news /wonk/wp/2015/04/22/youll-never-guess-the-worlds-fattest-country-and-no-its-not -the-u-s.

2. Amanda Gardner, "Another Study Links Western Diet to Heart, Health Risks," MedicineNet, January 18, 2022, https://www.medicinenet.com/script/main /art.asp?articlekey=86574.

3. Ed Yong, "Fat Cell Number Is Set in Childhood and Stays Constant in Adulthood," Science Blogs, May 4, 2008, http://scienceblogs.com/notrocket-science/2008/05/04/fat-cell-number-is-set-in-childhood-and-stays-constant-in-ad.

4. Myles S. Faith, Kelley S. Scanlon, Leann L. Birch, Lori A. Francis, and Bettylou Sherry, "Parent-Child Feeding Strategies and Their Relationships to Child Eating and Weight Status," *Obesity Research Journal* 12, no. 11 (December 2004): 1711–22, https://onlinelibrary.wiley.com/doi/abs/10.1038/oby.2004.212.

5. Ed Yong, "Fat Cell Number Is Set in Childhood and Stays Constant in Adulthood."

6. Obesity and Overweight," World Health Organization, June 9, 2021, https://www.who.int/news-room/fact-sheets/detail/obesity-and-overweight.

7. Alvina R. Kansra, Sinduja Lakkunarajah, M. Susan Jay. "Childhood and Adolescent Obesity: A Review." Frontiers in Pediatrics (Jan 2021), https://www.frontiersin.org/articles/10.3389/fped.2020.581461/full.

8. A. Miyawaki, J. S. Lee, and Y. Kobayashi, "Impact of the School Lunch Program on Overweight and Obesity among Junior High School Students: A Nationwide Study in Japan," *Journal of Public Health* 41, no. 2 (June 2019): 362–70, https://academic.oup.com/jpubhealth/article/41/2/362/5033367.

9. "Obesity and Overweight," World Health Organization, June 9, 2021, https://www.who.int/news-room/fact-sheets/detail/obesity-and-overweight.

10. Myles S. Faith, Kelley S. Scanlon, Leann L. Birch, Lori A. Francis, and Bettylou Sherry, "Parent-Child Feeding Strategies and Their Relationships to Child Eating and Weight Status," *Obesity Research Journal* 12, no. 11 (December 2004): 1711–22, https://onlinelibrary.wiley.com/doi/abs/10.1038/oby.2004.212.

11. Faith et al., "Parent-Child Feeding Strategies."

12. "Shojin Ryori: Japan's Sophisticated Buddhist Cuisine," Savor Japan, February 10, 2017, https://savorjapan.com/contents/more-to-savor/shojin-ryori-japans-sophisticated-buddhist-cuisine.

13. "Shojin Ryori: Japan's Sophisticated Buddhist Cuisine,"

14. Chico Harlan, "On Japan's School Lunch Menu: A Healthy Meal, Made From Scratch," *Washington Post*, January 26, 2013, https://www.washingtonpost.com/world/on-japans-school-lunch-menu-a-healthy-meal-made-from-scratch/2013/01/26/5f31d208-63a2-11e2-85f5-a8a9228e55e7_story.html.

15. Chico Harlan, "On Japan's School Lunch Menu: A Healthy Meal, Made From Scratch."

16. "Sleep and Disease Risk," Healthy Sleep, Division of Sleep Medicine, Harvard Medical School, December 18, 2007, http://healthysleep.med.harvard.edu/healthy/matters/consequences/sleep-and-disease-risk.

17. Karen Collins, "Help Ward Off Cancer with a Japanese Diet," NBC News, December 17, 2004, https://www.nbcnews.com/id/wbna6724128#.

18. Karen Collins, "Help Ward Off Cancer with a Japanese Diet."

19. Shoichiro Tsugane, "Why Has Japan Become the World's Most Long-Lived Country: Insights from a Food and Nutrition Perspective," *European Journal*

of Clinical Nutrition 75 (July 13, 2020): 921–28, https://www.nature.com/articles/ s41430-020-0677-5#.

20. Martin Juneau, "Why Do the Japanese Have the Highest Life Expectancy in the World?" Prevention Watch, March 9, 2021, https://observatoireprevention.org/ en/2021/03/09/why-do-the-japanese-have-the-highest-life-expectancy-in-the-world.

21. Juneau, "Why Do the Japanese Have the Highest Life Expectancy in the World?"

22. "Sleep and Disease Risk," Healthy Sleep.

23. Jianghong Liu, Ying Cui, Linda Li, Lezhou Wu, Alexandra Hanlon, Jennifer Pinto-Martin, Adrian Raine, and Joseph R. Hibbeln, "The Mediating Role of Sleep in the Fish Consumption–Cognitive Functioning Relationship: A Cohort Study," *Scientific Reports* 7 (2017): 1796, https://www.nature.com/articles/s41598 -017-17520-w.

24. Xian Jiang, Jiang Huang, Daqiang Song, Ru Deng, Jicheng Wei, and Zhou Zhang, "Increased Consumption of Fruit and Vegetables Is Related to a Reduced Risk of Cognitive Impairment and Dementia: Meta-Analysis," *Frontiers in Aging Neuroscience* 9 (February 7, 2017): 18, https://www.ncbi.nlm.nih.gov/pmc/articles /PMC5293796.

25. "Japan Shows Food Education Works," Medium, July 7, 2017, https:// medium.com/@BCFN_Foundation/japan-shows-food-education-works -6b7aa32cb809.

26. "Japan Shows Food Education Works," Medium.

27. Venturi Wang, "Using Chopsticks to Improve Kids Intelligence Quotient," Sooper Articles, November 30, 2011, https://www.sooperarticles.com/home-and -family-articles/using-chopsticks-improve-kids-intelligence-quotient-726050.html.

28. Henry Legere, *Raising Healthy Eaters* (Boston: Da Capo Lifelong Books, 2009), 51, 73.

29. Scott H. Sicherer, MD, "New Guidelines Detail Use of 'Infant Safe' Peanut to Prevent Allergy," AAP News, January 5, 2017, http://www.aappublications.org /news/2017/01/05/PeanutAllergy010517.

30. "The Pressure Is On to Keep Blood Pressure Down," Centers for Disease Control and Prevention, September 2014, https://www.cdc.gov/vitalsigns/children -sodium/index.html; "Healthy Kids 'Sweet Enough' without Added Sugars," Harvard School of Public Health, August 23, 2016, https://www.hsph.harvard.edu/ nutritionsource/2016/08/23/aha-added-sugar-limits-children.

31. Elizabeth Brown, "Different Words for Sugar on Food Labels," SFGate, December 6, 2018, https://healthyeating.sfgate.com/different-words-sugar-food -labels-8373.html.

32. Megan Clapp, Nadia Aurora, Lindsey Herrera, Manisha Bhatia, Emily Wilen, and Sarah Wakefield, "Gut Microbiota's Effect on Mental Health: The

Gut-Brain Axis," *Clinics and Practice* 7, no. 4 (September 15, 2017): 987, https://www.ncbi.nlm.nih.gov/pmc/articles/PMC5641835.

33. S. Lockyer and A. P. Nugent, "Health Properties of Resistant Starch," *Nutrition Bulletin* 42, no. 1 (March 2017): 10–41, https://doi.org/10.1111/nbu.12244.

CHAPTER 8

1. Kumiko Ninomiya, "Science of Umami Taste: Adaptation to Gastronomic Culture," *Flavour* 4, article 13 (January 26, 2015), https://flavourjournal.biomedcentral.com/articles/10.1186/2044-7248-4-13.

2. Kumiko Ninomiya, "Science of Umami Taste: Adaptation to Gastronomic Culture."

3. Kumiko Ninomiya, "Science of Umami Taste: Adaptation to Gastronomic Culture."

4. Kumiko Ninomiya, "Science of Umami Taste: Adaptation to Gastronomic Culture."

5. Janelle Weaver, "Fermented-Food Diet Increases Microbiome Diversity, Decreases Inflammatory Proteins, Study Finds," Stanford Medicine News Center, July 12, 2021, https://med.stanford.edu/news/all-news/2021/07/fermented-food-diet-increases-microbiome-diversity-lowers-inflammation.

CHAPTER 9

1. "Is Shinto a Religion?" BBC News, October 30, 2009, https://www.bbc.co.uk/religion/religions/shinto/beliefs/religion.shtml.

2. "Shintoism," United Religions Initiative, https://www.uri.org/kids/world-religions/shintoism.

3. "Shintoism," United Religions Initiative.

4. Moriyasu Ito, "Of Shinto and Japanese Culture," *Talks at Google*, July 7, 2016, https://www.youtube.com/watch?v=Ekl4urMCfEU.

5. Ito, "Of Shinto and Japanese Culture."

6. Pole Lee, Joseph Choi, and Ryan Sun, "Japanese Food Metaphysics," *Scholar Blogs*, May 11, 2020, https://scholarblogs.emory.edu/philosophyoffood/2020/05/11/japanese-food-metaphysics.

7. Lee, Choi, and Sun, "Japanese Food Metaphysics."

8. Lee, Choi, and Sun, "Japanese Food Metaphysics."

9. Lee, Choi, and Sun, "Japanese Food Metaphysics."

10. Elizabeth Scott, "What Is Spirituality?" Very Well Mind, November 27, 2020, https://www.verywellmind.com/how-spirituality-can-benefit-mental-and-physical-health-3144807.

11. Louise Delagran, "What Is Spirituality?" Taking Charge of your Health & Wellbeing, University of Michigan, https://www.takingcharge.csh.umn.edu/what-spirituality.

12. "Hatsumode: New Year's Tradition in Japan," *Japan Wonder Travel Blog*, December 22, 2021, https://blog.japanwondertravel.com/new-year-holidays-hatsumode-10261.

13. "Hatsumode: New Year's Tradition in Japan," *Japan Wonder Travel Blog*.

14. "Toshikoshi Soba: New Year's Eve Food," *Destination Japan*, August 3 [no year], https://www.hisgo.com/us/destination-japan/blog/toshikoshi_soba.html.

15. "Toshikoshi Soba: New Year's Eve Food," *Destination Japan*.

16. "Osechi, Otoso, and Kagami Mochi: New Year's Bento Box, Sake, and Mochi!" *Destination Japan*, August 8 [no year], https://www.hisgo.com/us/destination-japan/blog/osechi_otoso_and_kagami_mochi.html.

17. "Osechi, Otoso, and Kagami Mochi: New Year's Bento Box, Sake, and Mochi!" *Destination Japan*.

18. "Ozuni: Mochi Rice Cake Soup," *Destination Japan*, August 4 [no year], https://www.hisgo.com/us/destination-japan/blog/ozouni.html.

19. "First Meal," Cheer Up, September 21, 2016, https://english.cheerup.jp/article/3732?page=1&pager_auto=1.

20. "First Meal," Cheer Up.

21. "First Meal," Cheer Up.

22. "Shichi-Go-San," Nippon.com, November 9, 2015, https://www.nippon.com/en/features/jg00043.

23. "Shichi-Go-San," Nippon.com.

24. "Shichi-Go-San," Nippon.com.

25. "What the Heck Is Setsubun?" *GaijinPot Blog*, February 1, 2021, https://blog.gaijinpot.com/what-the-heck-is-setsubun.

26. "What the Heck Is Setsubun?" *GaijinPot Blog*.

27. Setsuko Yoshizuka, "Japanese Girls' Day or Hinamatsuri," The Spruce Eats, April 18, 2021, https://www.thespruceeats.com/hina-matsuri-2031037.

28. Setsuko Yoshizuka, "Japanese Girls' Day or Hinamatsuri."

29. Ai Faithy Perez, "Kodomo No Hi: A Guide to Children's Day in Japan," Savvy Tokyo, May 4, 2020, https://savvytokyo.com/kodomo-no-hi-guide-childrens-day-japan.

30. Ai Faithy Perez, "Kodomo No Hi: A Guide to Children's Day in Japan."

31. Ai Faithy Perez, "Kodomo No Hi: A Guide to Children's Day in Japan."

32. Ito, "Of Shinto and Japanese Culture.

Index

Index

About the Authors

Marie Akisawa is a registered dietitian and a chef. She has published four books on healthy cooking: 2014's *Beat Diabetes without Giving Up Gourmet Foods*, 2015's *Beat Diabetes with Low-Carb Cooking*, 2016's *117 Food Recipes for Beauty*, and 2017's *Almost Sugar-Free Cooking for Special Occasions*. She has published two books on supplements: 2003's *Supplement Magic,* and 2004's *How to Stay Beautiful and Healthy with Supplements*. Her newest book, published in 2022, *Diet Plan that Reversed Her Father's Diabetes Who's Still Working as an MD at the Age of 85*. She started cooking low-carb meals for her diabetic father from 2013 and successfully reversed his diabetes within a year. Her father is now 85 years old and still works as a medical doctor six days a week with no signs of complications. Armed with hundreds of original recipes, Marie opened a catering business called Marie's Low-Carb Foods in Japan, where she prepares meals which include healthy snacks, cakes, bread, pizzas, and also Japanese meals that are low in carbs and gluten free, and also provides consulting to restaurants.

Marie recently founded and is the chairwoman of the Japanese Nutritious Foods Association, where she and other nutritionists and doctors provide online seminars on nutrition. She is providing Shokuiku cooking classes for the Japanese children and their parents and hosts a weekly internet radio show, called "Marie's Room," to increase awareness of how Shokuiku—food education—influences longevity and disease prevention. She is an Institute for Integrative Nutrition-qualified health coach, a macrobiotic master, and was a finalist of the Miss Universe pageant, 1989 Kinki region, Japan. She is currently living in Japan.

YouTube:
https://youtube.com/channel/UCumoh62pYmYebrHkFWyea6w

Instagram:
@marieakisawa

Facebook:
https://www.facebook.com/marie.akisawa

Twitter:
@marie_akisawa

Motoko Kimura was raised by a mother who was a registered dietitian and a schoolteacher for over twenty-five years, Motoko's mother educated her daily on *Shokuiku* and which foods contained benefits for the body and our spiritual connection with food. As a result of being raised by the philosophy and education in this book, Motoko overcame being born weak and underweight as well as energy and attention issues as a young child. She was also never seriously ill or hospitalized as a child or an adult. Motoko turned her lifelong love of film and storytelling into a successful career as an author, and television and film producer. She is the best-selling author of *A Moment to Remember*, based on the television mini-series *Pure Soul*, which she created and produced. She then produced a film based on *Pure Soul* in 2004 in South Korea. The film became one of the biggest hits in all of Asia, grossing over $30 million, and is currently in preproduction for an American version of the film with Amazon. At age thirty-nine, Motoko felt the calling to become a mother, and after five years of fertility treatments, she was blessed with a beautiful baby boy at age forty-four. She is raising her son with the food education her mother gave her. Living half a year in Los Angeles and half a year in Tokyo, her now eight-year-old son has enjoyed an extremely healthy life.

Motoko realized she needed to write this book after splitting her time between America and Japan and hiring nannies from several different countries such as the Philippines, El Salvador, Mexico, and America. She found it shocking that none of them understood the importance of the right foods in a child's diet, and she had to educate each one of them. Traveling across the U.S., Motoko also noticed the vast difference in the way Americans view food versus her experience growing up in Japan. She realized if she could pass on the food education she received, the world could be a healthier place.

Twitter:
@yusukegen

Instagram:
@motoko.kimura

YouTube:
https://www.youtube.com/channel/UCkA5aMEvHoiep4d9ULXS5Mw

All illustrations in this book were created by Kaoru Takeuchi.